CHANGE
1 THING

CHANGE

1 THING

A DOCTOR'S 12 STEP PLAN FOR
PERMANENT WEIGHT LOSS, DISEASE
PREVENTION, AND A LIFETIME OF
INCREDIBLE HEALTH

Teresa Fuller, M.D. Ph.D

To order additional copies of this book, contact:
Xlibris Corporation
1-888-795-4274
www.Xlibris.com
Orders@Xlibris.com
114196

CONTENTS

This book is dedicated to my husband Julian, and our two sons Alexander and Steven, for being my biggest supporters, and providing me with the encouragement to get this book completed and published.

I also dedicate this book to my father who constantly told me "you can do anything you want if you want it bad enough."

ACKNOWLEDGEMENTS

I would like to acknowledge the many people who supported this Change 1 Thing Project. It began as a twelve month program that I implemented at New Hope Baptist Church in Baltimore, MD. Therefore, I would like to thank my Pastor, Dr. James Fuller and First Lady Ruth Fuller for welcoming this program at New Hope. I'd also like to thank the New Hope congregation for being willing participants in the program, and for challenging me to develop a new health challenge every month for our one year journey.

I'd also like to acknowledge my family who has patiently listened to me share these health insights with them week after week. You have all been a major encouragement for me to find well-researched information that will lead us to optimal health.

INTRODUCTION

All I remember thinking is "I'm too young for this." At the tender age of thirty-nine, I was too young to be hobbling around from an arthritis-like condition. I saw others of my peers complaining about various aches and pains, with the common consensus that this is what happens as you near the big four-zero. Really, am I not too young for this? It started insidiously, waking up in the mornings and having to limp around for the first thirty minutes or so until the pain in my feet gradually subsided. Then through various times of the day, the pain would return when I had been on my feet for a prolonged period. Ultimately, I went to a podiatrist to be diagnosed with plantar fasciitis. My podiatrist told me to wear special inserts in my shoes, practice stretching exercises, and take Motrin. If those things did not work, I might need steroid injections. Despite the inserts and the exercises, the pain continued. Was it the excess weight? I had gradually gone from 140 lbs to 170 lbs over the past few years, another inevitability I attributed to nearing the age of forty. Was it the long hours on my feet as a pediatric hospitalist? Not much I was able to do about that situation. So I suffered with the pain and started to come to a point of acceptance.

Then just two months before my fortieth birthday, I went on a cruise where I attended a presentation on healthy living. The presenter was a personal trainer and explained the importance of nutrition, exercise, and detoxification to a healthy life. During his presentation, he even talked about healing his arthritic hip condition using these natural strategies. For some reason, I knew that he was talking to me that now was the time for me to change my eating, start exercising, and detoxify my system. But how? What did I need to eat? What did I need to stop eating? And how would I detoxify? Did I need the expensive detoxification system that he recommended, or was there more to it? This burst of inspiration and these questions led me on a journey over the past year that has opened my eyes to the power of food for healing and the innate power of the body to heal itself when properly nourished.

I admit that I wasn't completely convinced at first. If you had asked me about my eating habits at that time, I would assess my diet as "not bad." In retrospect, it was sorely lacking in fresh fruits and vegetables and generously packed with refined foods and junk foods. After the presentation, I immediately changed my eating. As the saying goes, "I used the light that I had" and kept adjusting my eating habits as I learned better. But with just the first few changes that I made, which of course you will find in the pages of this book, I quickly lost the extra 30 lbs. They had taken a couple of years to pack on but only three months to melt off. But even more surprising than how quickly the weight fell off was the fact that I had also shed the painful foot condition. If you've ever gotten cured from a painful condition, you'll understand that I didn't even notice at first. But at some point, it occurred to me that I no longer limped around in the morning. What does that have to do with nutrition? As I was quickly learning, the anti-inflammatory foods that I was now eating cured that inflammatory condition of plantar fasciitis. The suffix—*itis* means "inflammation." Now, I'm a believer because not only have I studied the research about nutrition and disease, but I have experienced it for myself.

That's my story. What is yours? You're reading this book because you want solutions for your health issues. You want something that really works, not just for some people, but for you. You want to cut through all the confusing messages that you have heard in the news and on the Internet and get to the truth about healthy living.

As a physician, I have been asked by countless people how to lose weight and improve their health. In response, I created this system of twelve habits to give people a consistent and fail-proof method to achieve their health goals, and I have seen people get results. Unlike many programs that promise fast results using methods that can be sustained temporarily at best, the program outlined in this book recognizes that permanent results take time. Even more important, this program is designed to go beyond weight loss by instilling habits that have been scientifically proven to achieve disease prevention *and* disease reversal.

> *To listen is to lean in, softly, with a willingness* to be changed by what we hear *[emphasis mine]*.
>
> —Mark Nepo

I've been warned that asking people to change is a losing battle. Well, I don't believe that. I purposely included the word *change* in the title of this book because as you know, you can't do the same thing and expect different results. Something has to change.

In this book, I present simple, well-researched strategies that you can gradually incorporate into your life over a period of one year to achieve your health goals. I wrote this book for people who are frustrated with their failed attempts at permanent weight loss. This book takes you on a journey of adopting twelve habits that will result in permanent weight loss and markedly improved overall health. Since it takes twenty-one days to establish a new habit, the book is set up to give you one month to firmly establish one habit before tackling the next. In one year, you will have completely transformed your lifestyle.

How to Get the Most Out of This Book

- Take your time and incorporate these habits one by one. If you try to do it all at once, you may become overwhelmed and give up. Be patient with yourself. Remember that it took years to accumulate extra weight and unhealthy habits. Making changes one month at a time is a good pace.

- Use the tips for children. You'll find that each chapter contains helpful information on instilling these habits in your children's lifestyles as well as your own. As Dr. Hiromi Shinya says in his book *The Enzyme Factor*, "The older one gets, the harder it becomes to change one's habits. Moreover, habits that get imprinted in our minds while we are young often exercise a powerful influence over our entire lives. Therefore, it is important to imprint good habits on children as early as possible."

- Don't get discouraged. If you find that a few months in, you've slacked off on one of your newly developed healthy habits, just refocus on the habit and give yourself another thirty days to make it a part of your lifestyle.

Are you up to the challenge? Let's go!

January Challenge

I Will Drink My Optimal Amount of Water Every Day

How many times have you heard this, "You should drink eight glasses of water per day"? Probably more times than you can count. But at least 75% of Americans don't drink nearly that amount of water every day. Recently, after giving a talk on healthy living in which I emphasized the importance of drinking water, I was approached by a woman in the audience who told me that she hadn't had any water to drink in weeks! She was in the habit of satisfying her thirst with bottled green tea. Hopefully, after you've read this chapter, you'll know why that's not the proper way to hydrate your body.

Even though there is no recommended daily allowance for water, common consensus among health experts is that an adult should drink between two to three quarts of water per day. But since people vary in size, I like the more specific recommendation to drink the number of ounces of water equal to half your body weight in pounds daily. That means that if you weigh 150 pounds, you should drink seventy-five ounces of water per day—about nine and a half glasses. By the same token, a 40-pound child should drink twenty ounces or two and a half glasses of water per day.

Don't Be Fooled

I'm disturbed by the number of products that are labeled "water" these days. Look in the water or beverage section of the supermarket, and you will find a myriad of colorful and eye-catching concoctions labeled "water" in some way. However, the advantage of water to your body is in its purity. When the water is "enhanced" with flavors, colors, and sweeteners, whether artificial or natural, you've defeated the purpose. So here are some rules of thumb: If it has an ingredients list, it's not water. If it has a color to it, it's not water. And if it has a refreshingly sweet strawberry flavor to it, it's not water. One reason that it's important to drink plain water is to get your palate used to its bland taste and reduce your taste buds' demand for sugar.

Why Is Water Important

> *Water has many functions inside the human body, but the biggest function is to improve blood flow and promote metabolism. It also activates the intestinal bacteria flora and enzymes while excreting waste and toxins. Dioxins, pollutants, food additives and carcinogens are all flushed out of the body by good water. . . . For all these reasons people who do not drink enough good water will get sick more easily.*
>
> —Hiromi Shinya, *The Enzyme Factor*

Why do we need to drink so much water? Our bodies are 67% water! Water is critical to all bodily processes. A recent publication by Dr. Lawrence Armstrong indicates that a dehydration level of just 1.36% is enough to negatively affect concentration and mood and induce headaches. It is commonly known that a 5% dehydration status is enough to significantly interfere with the body's normal functioning. Consider these important benefits of water:

- Hydration boosts your immune system, which is your defense against disease-causing bacteria, viruses, parasites, and toxins.
- Hydration maintains an alkaline environment in your tissues. An alkaline environment is protective against numerous diseases, including the dreaded cancer.
- Hydration aids enzymatic processes in the body, which are critical to the variety of bodily functions.

Some people water their houseplants more than they do their own bodies! You are valuable; take care of yourself and properly hydrate your body.

—Don Colbert,
The Seven Pillars of Health

Is All Water Created Equal?

No. Although the most important thing you can do is drink your optimal amount of water every day, you don't want to drink just *any* water. Let's take a brief look at the problems associated with different types of water.

Tap water. I believe we are entitled to clean, safe drinking water from the tap. I am not alone in opinion, which is why groups like the Environmental Protection Agency (EPA) and the Environmental Working Group (EWG) are hard at work lobbying our government to clean up the nation's water. Unfortunately, tap water is polluted with numerous chemicals and pathogens (harmful bacteria, viruses, and parasites).

For example, chromium-6, also known as hexavalent chromium, has recently been in the news as a harmful chemical that has been found extensively in tap water. EWG found it in the drinking water of thirty-one out of thirty-five US cities. It is one of two hundred contaminants found in tap water that has no enforceable safety limit. Hexavalent chromium shows "clear evidence of carcinogenic activity" in lab animals and is likely to be a carcinogen in humans as well.

If you are a person who is proud to say that you take no prescribed medications, you might be dismayed at the number of medications you're exposed to in tap water. Pharmaceuticals such as antibiotics, sex hormones, and other prescription drugs are routinely found in tap water. They make their way into our water sources when their residues are flushed down the toilet in human waste products. These chemicals are not regulated and are not routinely tested for by water treatment plants. We do not even know the effects of the residues of these various pharmaceuticals on our bodies.

Did you hear the recent news about the government's decision to lower fluoride in tap water? After all these years, concerns about fluoride have finally been acknowledged. While fluoride has the benefit of reducing tooth decay, excess fluoride has quite a few side effects. The most common side effect is dental fluorosis, a condition of mottling and pitting of the tooth enamel that has been on the rise. Other important side effects of excess fluoride are skeletal fluorosis (brittle bones and increased fractures), neurotoxicity, and disruption of thyroid function.

Bottled water. At the risk of showing my age, I can remember the days when bottled water was first becoming popular. I was among the many who said something like "Water is free. Why would anyone pay for it?" Boy, were we wrong. Bottled water is now an almost-twenty-billion-dollar industry! With all the brands out there, can we even make any generalizations about bottled water?

Bottled water is not the best choice of water to regularly drink. First of all, you should know that one-third of all bottled water is simply tap water. (If you're skeptical, I didn't believe that when I first heard it either. But that is the case.) Also, a recent study by the EWG found frequent contamination of bottled water. Looking at ten brands of bottled water, they found an average of eight contaminants per brand, which included pharmaceuticals, heavy metals, and fertilizer residue among others. The plastic housing of the water may also be harmful. You've probably heard of BPA (bisphenol A), which is a component of plastic thought to increase breast cancer risk and reduce sperm counts.

Another significant problem with bottled water is that it is toxic to the environment. The process of creating the plastic bottles uses a huge amount of oil. And the bottles are polluting. Approximately 80% of the bottles end up in landfills.

A great alternative. Clean filtered water should be your choice. You can purchase a filter and carry your own bottle of water around to give yourself a regular supply of pure water. Not all water filters are created equally either. For example, distillers and reverse-osmosis filters are excellent at removing harmful chemicals and pathogens from your water, but they also remove beneficial minerals such as calcium, sodium, potassium, copper, manganese, iron, and magnesium. These filters may also create acidic water. For optimal health, you want to create a slightly alkaline environment in your body because an alkaline environment is most inhospitable to disease. Therefore, I recommend alkalinized filtered water.

> *You know the food pyramid. It is a chart designed by the National Institute [sic]of Health that prioritizes the foods we should eat . . . . Here is a prediction. The next redesign will have eight glasses of water at the pyramid's foundation.*
>
> —Steve Meyerowitz,
> *Water: The Ultimate Cure*

What You Can Expect From *This One Change*

You will have a decrease in the symptoms of dehydration. Dehydration leads to fatigue, headaches, backaches, and joint aches. As many as 75% of Americans are chronically dehydrated.

If you have problems with constipation, like 40% of Americans have, this one change will improve your regularity.

You will lose weight. Why? The average American drinks 10% of his or her daily caloric intake. By replacing sweetened beverages with plain water, you will be on your way to losing unwanted pounds.

Tips for Getting Your Optimal Daily Amount of Water

- Drink water when you wake up in the morning.
- Carry a thirty-two-ounce bottle (BPA free) of water with you and sip on water throughout the day.
- Drink water with your meals (but no more than eight ounces during the meal).

Tips for Helping Your Children Drink More Water

Start early. When your baby is old enough to expand fluid intake beyond milk, rather than giving him juice in a bottle, make it plain water. This will help the child develop a taste for it. By the way, if the baby is given a bottle when going to sleep, it should always be plain water to avoid later tooth decay.

For children, insist that they must drink a glass of water before they can have juice or other flavored beverage.

Have a water bottle designated for each child that they can easily access and sip on through the day.

Don't have alternatives. If you have sodas, juice, and other sugary drinks easily accessible to your children, they'll choose those options.

FAQs

Does it need to be water? Can't any fluid count?

Almost any other fluid brings with it an undesired ingredient. For example, fluids containing caffeine or alcohol are actually dehydrating. Juices contain sugar, which is an ingredient we need to significantly reduce in the average American diet. Diet drinks add chemicals to your body that have been shown to have harmful effects.

What if I don't like water?

Your body loves water. Your brain just hasn't caught up to that fact yet. Besides, water is an acquired taste if you have gotten used to drinking flavored beverages all the time. I guarantee you that after a short while of daily drinking your optimal amount of water, you will begin to love it. It becomes habit-forming!

What if water keeps me running to the bathroom?

I have good news! That effect only lasts for the first few days. Once your body adjusts, you will not have to urinate as frequently. However, you will need to urinate more frequently than you do now, and that is a sign that your body is properly cleansing and eliminating.

References

Armstrong LE, Ganio MS, Casa DJ, Lee EC, McDermott BP, Klau JF, Jimenez L, Le Bellego L, Chevillotte E, Lieberman HR. Mild dehydration affects mood in healthy young women. J Nutr. 2012 Feb; 142 (2): 382-8. Epub 2011 Dec 21.

Chromium-6 Is Widespread in US Tap Water: Cancer-causing chemical found in 89 percent of cities sampled: December 2010, http://www.ewg.org/chromium6-in-tap-water

Don Colbert, MD. *The Seven Pillars of Health.*(2007). Siloam, Lake Mary, FL

Meyerowitz, Steve, Water: The Ultimate Cure. Book Publishing Company, Summertown, TN 38483

Pharmaceuticals Pollute U.S. Tap Water: March 2008. http://www.ewg.org/node/26128

Shinya, Hiroma. The Enzyme Factor (2010) Council Oak Books, San Francisco & Tulsa

The Story of Bottled Water (2010); storyofstuff.org. http://www.youtube.com/watch?v=Se12y9hSOM0&feature=player_embedded

U.S. Catches Up with Science On Fluoride in Drinking Water: Jan 2011. EWG Public Affairs http://www.ewg.org/release/us-catches-science-fluoride-drinking-water.

FEBRUARY CHALLENGE

I Will Eat Seven to Nine Servings of Fruits and Vegetables Every Day

The news isn't that fruits and vegetables are good for you. It's that they are so good for you they could save your life.

—David Bjerklie,
Time Magazine **(October 20, 2003)**

Just out of curiosity, I did a Google search to find out how many vegetables exist in the world. As you can imagine, I couldn't find an exact answer, although I saw estimates of one thousand to several thousand. So let's be conservative and estimate that there are 1,500 different types of vegetables. Guess how many of that huge variety we Americans tend to eat? Four! That's right, 50% of American vegetable consumption consists of four veggies: canned tomatoes, white potatoes, iceberg lettuce, and onions.

With children, the situation appears to be even more dire. Half of all children consume less than one serving of fruit daily. In the vegetable category, the majority of their vegetable consumption is in the form of fried potatoes. The 2008 Feeding Infants and Toddlers Study found that among infants and toddlers, fruit and vegetable consumption is below recommended levels in each age group it studied.

You might be astonished to know how few fruits and vegetables Americans are eating these days. Or maybe you aren't since chances are that you're one of them. With the severe reduction in fruit and vegetable intake we are experiencing, is it any wonder that our health statistics are headed in the wrong direction?

Benefits of Fruits and Vegetables

Full of fiber. The USDA Dietary Guidelines for Americans recommends an intake of twenty-eight to thirty-five grams of fiber daily for adults. For children, fiber intake should be fourteen grams of fiber for every one thousand calories consumed. This can be achieved with a diet rich in fresh fruits, vegetables, whole grains, and legumes. The average American diet only provides about fifteen grams of fiber per day. Increased fiber content in your diet will help keep you regular and will stabilize your blood sugar. Increased fiber intake also helps you lose weight. Fiber keeps our digestive systems healthy and prevents constipation, a problem for at least 40% of Americans.

Full of antioxidants. What are antioxidants? Chemicals that inhibit oxidation. Oxidative stress is a state of imbalance in the body caused by the production of free radicals in excess of the body's ability to eliminate them. These free radicals react with critical components of cells, such as DNA, lipids, and proteins, and lead to cellular damage. Therefore, antioxidants are critical for neutralizing free radicals. Examples of antioxidants are vitamin C and beta-carotene, which are found in a variety of fruits and vegetables. These powerful chemicals reduce inflammation and oxidative stress in the body.

Full of vitamins and minerals. The American diet is deficient in numerous vitamins and minerals. The average American consumes a diet containing low levels of calcium, potassium, fiber, magnesium, vitamins A, C, and E to name a few. We know that low calcium levels contribute to bone disease. Magnesium deficiency is also associated with insufficient bone mineral density and increased levels of inflammation, which contributes to many diseases. Potassium is important for regulating blood pressure. In other words, each of these vitamins and minerals are crucial to proper functioning of our bodies.

High water content. It is estimated that 75% of Americans are dehydrated—chronically! Dehydration causes aches, pains, and fatigue. But more important than that, dehydration leads to reduced functioning of our immune system and other bodily processes. Not only do we drink too little water, but we also eat too much dry, dead food. Fruits and vegetables have high water content.

Special Considerations: Getting the Most out of Your Fruits and Vegetables

Think variety. Why do you think our earth is filled with such a variety of fruits and vegetables? They each have different micronutrients that our bodies need. For example, if I say beta-carotene, what do you think of? Carrots, most likely. If I say vitamin C, you probably think of oranges. Well, what if I say lutein, quercetin, or capsaicin? Ah, I bet I have you stumped on a few of those! A variety of fruits and vegetables will give your body an abundant supply of vitamins and minerals. It is unquestionably our lack of fruit and vegetable intake that has led to the widespread vitamin deficiencies that our society is facing.

Go for deep colors. The reds, yellows, blues, and purples of fruit are beautiful to look at, but the aesthetic quality is beside the point. These deep colors indicate their rich supply of antioxidants. Polyphenols, the most common of which are flavonoids, which are responsible for the deep color of fruits and vegetables, provide antioxidant properties to fruits and vegetables. You've heard that an apple a day keeps the doctor away? It turns out that the majority of flavonoids consumed by people in the United States are found in apples, as well as onions and tea.

Eat it raw. Many of the beneficial enzymes and nutrients provided by fruits and vegetables are destroyed or reduced by the cooking process. Therefore, eat most of your produce raw to benefit from their full power.

What You Can Expect from *This One Change*

Regularity and improved gastrointestinal health. Many Americans are constipated, and as a result, have unhealthy gastrointestinal systems. When stool hardens in the gut, it's not only painful, but it interferes with the gut's ability to properly break down foods, to absorb nutrients, and to perform its immune function. An adequate amount of fruits and vegetables provides the fiber necessary to keep you regular.

Weight loss. Fruits and vegetables are low-calorie, low-fat (or no-fat) foods that are filling. By eating seven to nine servings throughout the day, during meals and snacks, you will keep your blood sugar levels steady, which will keep your appetite under control. Moreover, using these power-packed foods as snacks will replace alternative high-calorie, nutrient-poor snack choices.

Increased energy and overall well-being. One of the reasons we experience energy lows during the day is because our blood sugar levels fluctuate. Fruits and vegetables gradually release glucose into our bloodstreams to avoid those large fluctuations, keeping our energy levels steady as well. You'll also experience increased overall well-being because the effects of the micronutrients from the fruits and vegetables will prevent and reverse disease in your body.

FAQ: Should I Eat Organic Fruits and Vegetables?

Organic fruits and vegetables are grown without the use of conventional pesticides, herbicides, and insecticides that are poisonous to our systems. Organic farmers use natural techniques for pest avoidance and soil enrichment, which are protective of the produce itself, as well as protective of the environment. Another great advantage of organic produce is that it contains higher amounts of vitamins and minerals compared to conventionally grown produce. Therefore, I strongly encourage the consumption of organic produce. By eating locally and seasonally, you can reduce the extra cost that is associated with organic produce.

However, since organic foods are more expensive, the Environmental Working Group has published a list of the most important fruits and vegetables that should be eaten from organic sources, which they call the "dirty dozen." They are the following:

celery	blueberries
peaches	nectarines
strawberries	bell peppers
apples	spinach
cherries	potatoes
kale (collard greens)	grapes (imported)

Strategies for Eating More Fruits and Vegetables

Eat fruit with breakfast, like a serving of berries in your oatmeal. You can keep a supply of dried fruit on hand to mix into your breakfast cereal.

- Have a hearty salad with lunch or even for lunch. Add a vegetable soup, and you have at least three or four servings at lunch.
- Make a smoothie of blended-up fruits and vegetables to go with your dinner meal. Kids love smoothies, and you can easily hide vegetables in a smoothie without kids knowing it!
- Juice your fruits and vegetables with a quality juicer; you can find loads of fresh juice recipe ideas on the Internet.
- Eat a serving of raw fruit or vegetables as snacks between breakfast and lunch and dinner. It takes a bit of planning, but pack a bag of raw carrots and a pear or apple to make it convenient. That will not only boost your servings of fruit and veggies but will also keep you from turning to the vending machine.

Tips for Helping Your Children Eat More Fruits and Vegetables

Smoothies are a tasty way for children to get fresh fruits and vegetables. Most children love fresh or frozen smoothies, and you can vary them with all sorts of different fruits. And you can hide bland-tasting vegetables in smoothies as well. Be sure to make your own smoothies so that they have no added sugars or preservatives.

Use dips. I was surprised how much more my child was willing to eat raw vegetables using a salad dressing to dip them in.

Have fruits and vegetables available for snacks when your kids are most hungry. My son often eats bananas after school because they're sitting out on the table. Have them available during car rides with your children so that when they say, "I'm hungry," you can hand them a bunch of grapes or some slices of an orange.

A Different Perspective on Seafood

An often overlooked source of plant-based nutrition is sea vegetation. Kelp, for example, is an abundant source of vitamins and minerals. In fact, it's an excellent source of iodine, which is a necessary mineral for thyroid function. Spirulina, an alga, is considered by many to be a superfood. It supplies the essential fatty acid called gamma linolenic acid, which helps improve circulation and nerve conduction. Spirulina is also an excellent source of antioxidants.

Don't Forget to Continue your:

Continue your January habit of drinking at least eight glasses of water every day!

References

Increasing total fiber intake reduces risk of weight and fat gains in women.—Tucker LA—*J Nutr*—01-MAR-2009; 139 (3): 576-81. DOI: 10.3945/jn.108.096685

BRIEFEL, R, New Findings from the Feeding Infants and Toddlers Study: Data to Inform Action. December 2010, Supplement to the Journal of the American Dietetic Association EWG's Shopper's Guide to Pesticides

Holt, E., Steffen, L., Basu, S., Steinberger, J., Ross, J., Ping Hong, C., Sinaiko, A.

Fruit and Vegetable Consumption and Its Relation to Markers of Inflammation and Oxidative Stress in Adolescents. Journal of the American Dietetic Association—Volume 109, Issue 3 (March 2009) DOI: 10.1016/j.jada.2008.11.036

Logan, A. The Brain Diet. (2006). Nashville, TN, Cumberland House Publishing.

Murakami K, Dietary fiber intake, dietary glycemic index and load, and body mass index: a cross-sectional study of 3931 Japanese women aged 18-20 years. *Eur J Clin Nutr*—01-AUG-2007; 61 (8): 986-95

Position of the American Dietetic Association: Health Implications of Dietary Fiber Journal of the American Dietetic Association—Volume 108, Issue 10 (October 2008)—DOI: 10.1016/j.jada.2008.08.007

USDA Dietary Guidelines for Americans 2010

MARCH CHALLENGE

I Will Get the White Out and Go Whole

Refined sounds like such a nice word, doesn't it? But when it comes to food, *refined* means "severely denuded of nutrients, texture, and power." One thing I want to convince you of in this book is that food is powerful for healing. But when we start to process it, we strip it of its natural power.

"Get the white out" refers to getting the refined foods out of your diet. Refined foods are generally white: they include white flour, sugar, and white rice. What's wrong with these foods? First of all, the refining process strips them of the many nutrients that they had in their natural state. White flour is a stripped form of whole wheat flour, just as white rice is a stripped form of brown rice. They've also been stripped of fiber. Not only are they devoid of nutrients, but they add inflammation to your body. Inflammation is at the root of numerous diseases, including asthma, arthritis, and heart disease!

So how many servings of whole grains are you getting every day? If you're an average American, you are eating less than one serving of whole grains per day. But you should eat at least three servings per day if you are over nine years of age and at least two servings per day for children between the ages of four and eight years.

Health Benefits from Whole Grains

Full of fiber. Whole grain cereals are an excellent source of fiber. As complex carbohydrates, they stabilize blood sugar, preventing the swings of blood sugar that cause fat storage and cravings. Whole grains have been shown to protect against diabetes, cancer, constipation, diverticular disease, and various inflammatory disorders. Fiber is also a great detoxifier, helping the body rid itself of the numerous toxins it encounters daily. Fiber supports the beneficial bacteria in the gut.

Vitamins and minerals. Many micronutrients and trace minerals are found in these rich plant sources, such as selenium, a powerful antioxidant; zinc, an immune system booster; magnesium; calcium; iron; and folate. Whole grains are also a rich source of the B vitamins: thiamin, niacin, riboflavin, and panthothenic acid. B vitamins are critical to energy production in your body.

Good source of antioxidants. As plant sources, these foods also provide antioxidants to protect your body against inflammation and oxidative stress.

Special Considerations: What about Gluten Intolerance?

Gluten is a protein that is found in some grain products. It turns out that many people have gluten intolerance, meaning that they don't properly break down this protein. The severe form of gluten intolerance is a disease called celiac disease, which often causes diarrhea and poor weight gain in children. However, some people have a much more subtle form of gluten intolerance, which causes digestive problems. Whole grains that contain gluten include wheat, barley, rye, and some oats. If you are gluten intolerant, or suspect that you may be, these grains should be avoided.

What You Can Expect from *This One Change*

Weight loss. A major contributor to obesity is the excess sugar that we take in, whether it's from actual table sugar or from foods that are quickly broken down to sugar, like white flour. Whole grains slowly and steadily release glucose into your bloodstream, keeping your appetite under control. Also, when you eat whole foods instead of refined, you eat less because whole foods are bulkier and, therefore, filling. Studies have shown a positive correlation between increased fiber intake and both weight and fat loss.

Regularity. By replacing refined foods with whole, fiber-rich foods, we decrease constipation. At least 40% of Americans are chronically constipated because our diets are low in fiber.

Decreased risk of heart disease and stroke. Refined foods are inflammatory. And one by-product of inflammation is hardening of the arteries, which leads to high blood pressure (making your heart work harder) and poor blood circulation to vital organs (like the heart and brain). Studies have shown that consumption of whole grains is associated with a lower risk of the following diseases:

- Hypertension
- Insulin sensitivity
- Type 2 diabetes
- Metabolic syndrome
- Obesity
- Some types of cancers

Feeling better. When your blood sugar levels are steady, you maintain a steady energy level. Decreased inflammation will cause an improvement in the aches and pains that you may be chronically dealing with.

Tips:

- Replace white rice with brown rice.
- Replace white bread with whole grain bread. Ezekiel bread is the king of whole grain breads. It's composed of a variety of whole grains and even provides a good amount of protein.
- Stop the sugar. Learn to sweeten your foods with fresh fruit, fresh fruit juice, and even small amounts of natural sweeteners like grade B maple syrup, molasses, or raw honey.

Tip for Getting Kids to Eat More Whole Grains

Children are creatures of habit. White foods should be a foreign food in your house. Make sure your kids know that bread and rice are brown.

When I switched to brown rice, my children rebelled. So I had to experiment a bit to make it more palatable. When I made fried brown rice seasoned with soy sauce, my older son loved it. When I made a coconut brown rice, my younger son loved it. Use the Internet for its vast repository of recipes for whole grains.

Desserts are good candidates for whole grains. For example, brown rice pudding or brown rice crispy treats. Use them in moderation, of course, to minimize sugar intake, but do use them.

And don't forget to continue your

January habit of drinking an optimal amount of water per day (one-half of your weight in ounces of water per day) and

February habit of eating seven to nine servings of fruit and vegetables per day.

References

Logan, A. The Brain Diet. (2006). Nashville, TN, Cumberland House Publishing.

O'Neil, C., Nicklas, T., Zanovec, M., Cho, S. Whole-grain consumption is associated with diet quality and nutrient intake in adults: the national health and nutrition examination survey, 1999-2004. The Journal of the American Dietetic Association. October 2010 Vol 110: 1461-1468

Tucker, LA. Increasing total fiber intake reduces risk of weight and fat gains in women. *J Nutr*—01-MAR-2009; 139 (3): 576-81

USDA Dietary Guidelines for Americans 2010

Zanovec, M., O'Neil, C., Cho, S., Kleinman, R., Nicklas, T. Relationship between whole grain and fiber consumptions and body weight measures among 6—to 18-year-olds. J Pediatr 2010; 157: 578-83).

APRIL CHALLENGE

I Will Exercise for Thirty Minutes at least Five Times per Week

The January 2012 issue of the *AARP Bulletin* bears this headline: "Sitting Is the New Smoking." As growing evidence shows that prolonged sitting increases the risk of obesity, as well as the risk of diseases such as cancer, diabetes, and early death, it is becoming more apparent that a sedentary lifestyle is "hazardous to your health".

Many of our work-related and leisurely activities now involve prolonged sitting—usually in front of a screen of some sort. For example, remember when you had to go to the library and search the shelves for information or to borrow books? Now, you can surf the Internet or download to your e-reader from the comfort of your chair. Remember hanging clothes to dry? You now likely use an electric dryer. Going grocery shopping? Now more people are choosing the convenience of delivery. The examples abound.

However, these labor-saving devices have not increased our time. Americans are busier than ever. In fact, the most common reason people give for not exercising is lack of time. I think another major reason is lack of the fun factor. Exercise often feels like one more thing to cross off the "to do" list. In other words, "I have to go to the gym" or "I have to do thirty minutes on the treadmill."

It's a chore. But when you were a child, it was simply play, and no one had to force you to do it.

How Well Are We Moving?

According to the CDC, less than 50% of adults meet the guidelines for regular aerobic activity. Regarding muscle strengthening exercise, less than 25% of adults meet the guidelines. Yet muscle building is an efficient way to boost weight loss. Among youth, the numbers are not much better. Only about 50% of adolescents are vigorously active on a regular basis.

So How Much Exercise Do We Need?

Children and adolescents should get sixty minutes of vigorous exercise per day. In addition to aerobics, the exercise should include muscle-strengthening activities, such as push-ups or climbing activities, and bone-strengthening activities, such as jumping rope or running three times per week.

Adults should practice a mixture of moderate and vigorous exercise for at least 150 minutes per week (which averages to 30 minutes five days per week) and muscle-strengthening exercises at least two days per week. Good muscle-building activities for adults can include weight lifting, using resistance bands, or yoga.

Benefits of Exercise

Exercise benefits every system in our bodies and produces a myriad of benefits for adults and children. Let's take a look at some of these benefits.

Exercise reduces obesity. This is not hard to believe, is it? And since we know that obesity increases the risk for a variety of diseases such as heart disease, type 2 diabetes, bone disease, cancer, liver disease, and others, then exercise will reduce the likelihood of these diseases as well.

Exercise is great for the heart. Exercise has been shown to reduce blood pressure. And by doing so, it reduces the risk for stroke and coronary artery disease. Studies have shown as much as a 31% reduction in cardiovascular disease among people who regularly exercise.

Exercise reduces cancer. One-third of the cases of breast, colon, and kidney cancer are attributed to obesity and lack of physical activity. Exercise can, therefore, reduce your risk of these diseases. For example, studies have shown that physical activity can reduce breast cancer risk by as much as 30% to 40%.

Exercise reduces bone disease. Obesity is a primary risk factor for osteoarthritis. In women who were overweight, as measured by a body mass index of greater than 25, a loss of just 5.1 kg (about 10 lbs) cut the risk of osteoarthritis by 50%. Exercise also has a positive effect on bone mineral density and strength, thereby reducing the risk of osteoporosis.

Exercise improves mental health. Exercise reduces depressive symptoms and reduces anxiety in both adults and children. Studies have shown that exercise can be as effective as antidepressant medication. It makes sense because exercise regulates neurotransmitter release in the brain, most notably dopamine and serotonin. These are the same neurotransmitters targeted by the most common antidepressant medications on the market. Exercise is also associated with improved self-esteem and improved behavior in children.

What about attention deficit hyperactivity disorder (ADHD), that condition characterized by impulsivity, inattention, and hyperactivity? Exercise can reduce symptoms of ADHD. A recent study led by Catherine Davis, a clinical health psychologist at the Georgia Prevention Institute at Georgia Health Sciences University in Augusta, showed that exercise increased activity in the executive-functioning area of the brain. Executive functioning includes self-control, planning, reasoning, and abstract thought. Self-control and planning of course are a problem in ADHD.

Exercise is great for the brain. Studies have shown that physical activity enhances memory and learning, reasoning, attention, problem solving, and intelligence testing. Exercise also promotes neurogenesis, which is the production of new nerve cells, and protects the nervous system from injury and neurodegenerative disease. Want to decrease your risk of dementia in half? Exercise does this. Your risk of Alzheimer's disease can be reduced by as much as 60% by exercise! Exercise also increases brain volume in areas implicated in executive processing. By the way, by reducing the risk of diabetes, high blood pressure, and cardiovascular disease, which all have a negative effect on brain function, exercise further protects the brain.

One way that exercise improves brain function is simply through enhanced blood flow. Blood removes waste products that accumulate in the brain. Along with that increased blood flow comes oxygen. The oxygen acts as a scavenger of free radicals, which damage brain cells.

Exercise slows aging. Studies indicate that the presence or absence of a sedentary lifestyle is among the greatest predictors of aging.

Ideas for Making It Happen

- Take a thirty-minute walk. Walking may be the best exercise you can do; it's aerobic, and it strengthens the bones. Outdoor walking can have the added benefits of interesting scenery, fresh air, and changing terrain, such as hills. Make sure your pace is fast enough to get your heart rate up.
- Put on some good music and simply dance or step in your living room for thirty minutes. Remember, exercise should be fun, and so simply dancing to music that lifts your

mood is a great activity. Remember to "dance like no one's watching!"

- Record an exercise program from the television and simply follow the routine. (It's like having a free personal trainer!)
- Break it up if needed. You can exercise for ten minutes at a time, three times per day for just as much benefit as a thirty-minute stretch.
- Make a conscious effort to move more even when you're not exercising. If you have a sedentary job, get up and move around for at least five minutes every hour.

Tips for Kids

Exercise is natural for young kids. How often do we envy their boundless energy? But they need a conducive environment to encourage those natural tendencies. Here are a few tips:

Remember to make it fun. Most kids aren't going to want to walk on a treadmill for thirty minutes. (In fact, neither do I.) That's boring. A great strategy for getting kids moving is to simply let them play outside. They can play ball, ride their bikes (with a helmet, of course), or climb trees. Be willing to get out there with them to encourage them.

Know that kids love to mimic you. I have fond memories of doing jumping jacks and jogging in place alongside my dad in the basement. He exercised every day (and still does in his late eighties). I didn't know it was exercise; it was just fun doing what he did.

Beware of the screen. Our technology-saturated environment strongly tempts children to sit in front of the television or sit and play video games for hours. First of all, as the American Academy of Pediatrics recommends, limit screen time to two hours per day for children over two years of age (and zero screen time for younger children). But don't let them mope; get them out exercising.

FAQs

What if I can't exercise because of a physical condition (e.g., arthritis, heart disease)?

Exercise is so versatile. People with illnesses can engage in exercises that fit their limitations, and they will often benefit from the effort. Discuss options with your physician or a personal trainer.

What if I don't have time to exercise?

I completely empathize with people who have busy schedules and find it challenging to fit in exercise. But here's a quote that reminds me of how critical it is to make time for exercise. "Those who think they have not time for bodily exercise will sooner or later have to find time for illness," as stated by Edward Stanley, former prime minister of the United Kingdom.

How Schools Are Working Against Themselves

Did you know that 50% of high schools don't provide physical education classes at all? Schools have started devaluing physical education and sacrificing it to make more room for academics. This is a grave error. Students do better academically when they get regular exercise.

A recent review of fourteen studies released by the Archives of Pediatrics and Adolescent Medicine in January 2012 "found strong evidence of a significant positive relationship between physical activity and academic performance." It is postulated that the increased flow of blood and oxygen to the brain may be the reason behind this trend.

One great study that showed this connection was published by Dr. Catherine Davis at the Georgia Health Sciences University. The study was performed on 171 children from age seven to eleven years who were assigned to exercise twenty minutes, forty minutes, or none at all every day after school. The kids were evaluated using cognitive tests and MRI brain scans. Kids who exercised had increased activity in the executive-functioning area of the brain (self-control, planning, reasoning, and abstract thought), in the prefrontal cortex (complex thinking and social behavior), and increased cognitive ability in math. Kids who exercised forty minutes per day had higher gains than those who exercised twenty minutes per day.

Some schools have found this same trend. For example, in Naperville District of Illinois, a concept called Zero Hour PE was introduced, which is a physical education course that occurs prior to the start of the school day. Academically, this district consistently ranks among the top ten in the state of Illinois and showed outstanding performance on standardized science and math testing.

So your challenge this month is to get moving and make exercise a daily habit or at least five days a week!

And don't forget to continue your

January habit of drinking your optimal amount of water per day (one-half of your weight in ounces of water per day),

February habit of eating seven to nine servings of fruit and vegetables per day, and

March habit of replacing refined white foods with whole grains.

References

Archives of Pediatrics & Adolescent Medicine, news release, Jan 2, 2012

Davis CL Exercise improves executive function and achievement and alters brain activation in overweight children: a randomized, controlled trial.—*Health Psychol*—01-JAN-2011; 30 (1): 91-8

Exercise builds brain health: key roles of growth factor cascades and inflammation.—Cotman CW—*Trends Neurosci*—01-SEP-2007; 30 (9): 464-72

Exercise is brain food: the effects of physical activity on cognitive function.—Ploughman M—*Dev Neurorehabil*—01-JUL-2008; 11 (3): 236-40

Exercise: the Data on its Role in Health, Mental Health, Disease Prevention, and Productivity. Primary Care: Clinics in Office Practice—Volume 35, Issue 4 (December 2008)

McCall, A., and Raj, R. Exercise for prevention of obesity and diabetes in children and adolescents. Clin. Sports Med 28 (2009) 393-421.

Medina, John, Brain Rules: 12 Principles for Surviving and Thriving at Work, Home and School. (2008). Pear Press. Seattle Washington.

Pope, E. Sitting: Hazardous to your health. AARP Bulletin, Jan-Feb 2012, Vol 53, No. 1, p 28.

Ratey, J., Hagerman, E. Spark: The revolutionary new science of exercise and the brain. (2008). Little, Brown and Company, New York, NY

Woods, J., Vieira, V., Keylock, T. Exercise, inflammation and innate immunity. Immunol Allergy Clin N Am 29 (2009) 381-393. http://www.cdc.gov/nchs/fastats/exercise.htm

MAY CHALLENGE

I Will Start to Detoxify My System Daily

A few years ago, my husband and I went on a trip to the Bahamas. My husband, Julian, was suffering from his seasonal allergies at the time and so was manifesting the symptoms of frequent sneezing, congestion, headaches, and fatigue. When we arrived to Freeport that evening, Julian chose to turn in early because he felt so miserable. I feared that this would be one of our least favorite vacations. However, the next morning, he arose fully restored and symptom-free. He did not have a single recurrence of allergy symptoms during our entire stay in the Bahamas. When we returned to Baltimore International Airport, shortly after deplaning, Julian immediately developed sneezing, congestion, and headache. It was the most dramatic illustration that I have seen of how toxic our environment is!

We are surrounded by a toxic environment. Toxins abound in our foods, water, and air in the form of pesticides, heavy metals, air pollutants, harsh cleaning products, etc. We can't avoid many of these toxins, and therefore, we need to be proactive in protecting our bodies against the harmful effects of these agents.

Most people think of detoxification as a process to take the body through every few months or once a year. Some people also equate detoxification with colon cleansing. While there is a place for these practices, I would like you to think of detoxification as your body carries it out, and that is as a continuous process that occurs day in and day out. Therefore, the detoxification plan that I recommend is simply supporting our bodies' natural detoxification system by (1) not overwhelming it with avoidable toxins and (2) using foods that support that system. Detoxification should not be an infrequent process any more than bathing your body is. Therefore, the following is a plan for you to detoxify your system daily.

Stop Toxin Intake!

The first thing we must do to detoxify is to *stop taking avoidable toxins into our systems.* The biggest offenders are cigarette smoke, alcohol, and drugs. But there are many other substances that we use regularly that are also toxic to our systems.

Sugar, for example, causes inflammation in our bodies. Excessive sugar wreaks havoc on our systems by causing rapid spikes in insulin levels, feeding yeast, and causing oxidative stress. It is also addictive to the point that some government agencies are seriously discussing regulating it!

Excessive caffeine stresses our bodies through elevated blood pressure and heart rate. Caffeine intake has increased substantially, especially in children and adolescents. So-called energy drinks are being promoted as the answer to fatigue. Recently, one leading energy drink has started marketing its product for daily use. And as this caffeine consumption increases, so do the caffeine overdoses as manifested by increased numbers of adults and children presenting to the ER with symptoms of caffeine overdose, such as rapid heart rate and palpitations.

Artificial sugars, flavors, and colors in many snack foods are also inflammatory and linked to increased frequency of mental health problems, such as anxiety and reduced memory. Some of these chemicals are also associated with other negative health consequences such as headaches, cardiac disease, and cancers.

Animal fat. Animals, including humans, store toxins in the fat cells. Therefore, when you eat animal fat, you are exposing your body to excessive toxins. Although lean meat reduces your animal fat intake, you are still consuming a significant amount of fat embedded in the meat. The best way to reduce animal fat exposure is to reduce your meat intake.

Plastics. Bisphenol A (BPA), styrene, phthalates, and other plastic products have all been shown to interfere with our bodies' natural processing, especially hormone functioning.

Heavy metals, such as lead, aluminum, and mercury, are toxic to our brains and other organs. They have been associated with neurologic dysfunction, behavioral effects, decreased sperm counts, spontaneous abortions, and prematurity. They may be contributing factors to the pediatric disorders of autism and ADHD.

Pesticides are everywhere; they're used widely in farming, thus contaminating our foods. Many people also use them for personal lawn care, gardening, and household pest control. Elevated levels of pesticides in our bodies are associated with a variety of neurotoxic effects, such as cognitive functioning, behavioral disturbance, and even seizures.

So the first step to detoxification is to stop or reduce eating foods and using products that contain these toxic chemicals.

Eat Detoxifying Foods

Dr. Alan Logan, author of *The Brain Diet,* has rightly said, "Your ability to detoxify is only as good as the quality of your diet." You need to fill your diet with foods that support the liver and gastrointestinal tracts, which are our bodies' main detoxification organs. Take a look at the following:

- Fiber binds toxic chemicals and removes them from the body through the gastrointestinal tract. It also promotes growth of "good bacteria" in the gut. Therefore, eat fiber-rich foods, such as brown rice, barley, beans, fruits, and vegetables.
- The cruciferous vegetables, which include cabbage, broccoli, brussels sprouts, and cauliflower, support the liver's detoxification process.
- Organic foods are foods grown or raised without use of hormones, pesticides, and other harmful chemicals. I realize these foods are more expensive, but they are worth it in the long run. The best foods to eat organically include beef and fruits and vegetables with thin or edible skins, such as apples, pears, and berries.

Decrease the Toxins in Your Personal Space!

Obtain a healthy weight. Again, toxins get stored in the fat cells of the body. By losing excess weight, you give your body less opportunity to hang on to toxic chemicals.

Decrease your pesticide exposure. Remove your shoes when entering your house to avoid tracking pesticides into the various rooms. Consider alternative, eco-friendly pest reduction products for your lawn and garden. And eat organic fruits and vegetables when possible, especially those that are on the "dirty dozen" list (see chapter 2).

Reduce your plastic load. Avoid microwaving or storing foods in plastic. Many frozen foods are now placed in plastic trays for easy microwaving, but that's a bad idea. Heating these foods in plastic containers allows the plastic to leach into the foods. Also, canned foods are often lined with plastic. Avoid canned items, and instead, choose glass-stored fruits and vegetables. (Of course, better yet, use fresh or frozen fruits and vegetables.) Pay attention to the number on the plastic bottles: Numbers 1 and 2 are best. Numbers 3, 6, and 7 increase your exposure to PVC, styrene, and BPA respectively.

Consider fasting. Water or juice fasting is an excellent strategy for ridding the body of toxins. Juice fasting involves drinking fresh juices that you make in a juicer at home (not store-bought juices). The load of antioxidant substances that you ingest from fresh juices will support your body's natural detoxification system. Before fasting, make sure that you get guidance from your health provider.

What You Can Expect from *This One Change*

Increased energy. The accumulation of toxic materials causes fatigue and interferes with your body's metabolism.

Weight loss. By eating detoxifying foods, including a diet high in fiber and loaded with detoxifying vegetables, you will naturally lose excess weight.

Reduced aches and pains. Inflammatory foods like sugar and artificial food additives cause inflammation in the body, which leads to a myriad of symptoms including musculoskeletal pain; cleaning these out of your diet will reduce these symptoms.

Detoxification Concerns for Children

Children are more vulnerable to the toxins in our environment than we are as adults for several reasons:

- Children have a greater surface-area-to-body-mass ratio, thus increasing chances of skin absorption.
- Children eat more food and drink more water per unit of body weight than adults do.

- Children have greater respiratory minute ventilation, meaning inspired air per unit time adjusting for weight.

Because of these factors, children have a higher chance of absorbing, ingesting, and inhaling toxins. Even more concerning is the fact that children experience a significant exposure to chemicals long before they are even born. A small study that looked at the umbilical cord blood of ten newborns found a total of 287 chemicals in the blood samples, including mercury, industrial by-products, and pesticides. Some of these chemicals are associated with brain toxicity, hormone dysfunction, and increased risk of cancer. Therefore, it is imperative that pregnant women avoid toxins in food and cooking and storage containers and maintain a healthy pregnancy weight.

So focus this month on incorporating these strategies to reduce the toxic load in your body. *Are you up to the challenge?*

Don't forget to continue your

January habit of drinking your optimal amount of water per day (one-half of your weight in ounces of water per day),

February habit of eating seven to nine servings of fruit and vegetables per day,

March habit of replacing refined white foods with whole grains, and

April habit of exercising for at least thirty minutes five times per week.

References

Bisphenol A (BPA) Information for Parents: US Department of Health and Human Services: http://www.hhs.gov/safety/bpa/

Houlihan et al "Body Burden: The Pollution in Newborns," Environmental Working Group, July 14, 2005

Seifert SM, Schaechter JL, Hershorin ER, Lipshultz SE. Health effects of energy drinks on children, adolescents, and young adults. Pediatrics. 2011 Mar; 127 (3): 511-28. Epub 2011 Feb 14. Review The National Institute of Environmental Health Sciences. Since You Asked—Bisphenol A (BPA): Questions and Answers about Bisphenol A http://www.niehs.nih.gov/news/sya/sya-bpa/

June Challenge

I Will Sleep for Seven to Eight Hours Every Night

Some years ago, when I was in residency training, I was desperately trying to learn to survive on minimal sleep. I came across a book called *The Sleep Solution*, which taught that anybody could train their bodies to get used to five or fewer hours of sleep. Eureka! I thought this was the answer to my dilemma. Well, now that I'm older and wiser, I know better. Sure, you can survive on a few hours of sleep every night. But it's not *healthy*. In fact, it's detrimental to your health, especially your brain health. And it's counterproductive to any weight loss plan.

Sleep is a serious problem in this society these days! Almost a quarter of Americans report having insomnia every night or most nights. An estimated forty-seven million Americans have a sleep disorder that interferes with daily functioning. Sleeping aids are prescribed and sold at record numbers, and now they are increasingly used by children and adolescents.

I think a major contributing factor to the increase in sleep deprivation is that sleep is severely undervalued in our society. We value activity and busyness. There aren't enough hours in a day, so who has time for sleep? We think sleep is a waste of precious time that should be used for more important pursuits. Therefore, we wear our droopy eyes and frequent yawns as badges of honor, proudly indicating how busy (read *important*) we are.

By the end of this chapter, I hope you realize that a good night's sleep is just as essential to optimal health as proper nutrition and exercise.

Why Is Sleep Important?

[S]leep is the golden chain that ties health and our bodies together.

—Thomas Dekker

- Sleep is critical to brain function. Experiments show that sleep deprivation causes impairment of performance, concentration, vigilance, and memory. Sleep is believed to be critical to the formation of new memories. New research is showing that chronic sleep deprivation can have permanent effects on memory and brain cell connectivity. The impairment of sleep deprivation on reaction time and cognition is profound. According to Charles Czeisler, Professor of Sleep Medicine at Harvard Business School, "We now know that 24 hours without sleep or a week of sleeping four or five hours a night induces an impairment equivalent to a blood alcohol level of 0.1%." That is higher than the legally drunk blood alcohol level of 0.08%!

- Studies show a strong link between inadequate sleep and obesity. That may sound counterintuitive, but the trend has been shown in both kids and adults. Epidemiologic studies show that during the period of escalating obesity rates in children, nocturnal sleep duration has declined. This does not prove that reduced sleep causes obesity, but there appears to be a link. Other studies have found correlations between sleep restriction and hormonal levels that influence weight gain. Moreover, sleep deprivation tends to cause an increased craving for simple carbohydrates, which may be another mechanism that leads to weight gain.

- Sleep deprivation suppresses the immune system. Lack of sleep may be a powerful contributor to chronic diseases and upper respiratory infections by impairing the body's immune response.

- Abnormal sleep duration increases your risk for type 2 diabetes. A study published in *Diabetes Care* found that adults who slept for less than five hours per night or greater than eight hours per night had increased incidence of type 2 diabetes. A survey study released in 2010 also associated these abnormally short or long sleep durations with hypertension and heart disease.

Given how critical sleep is for regulating brain, hormonal, and immune function to name a few, can't we see that depriving our bodies of sleep for the sake of productivity is counterproductive?

Special Considerations

How much sleep is enough? Depends on your age. Adults should get seven to eight hours of sleep per night. But children need more sleep. Children between the ages of two and six years should sleep for ten to twelve hours per day; seven—to thirteen-year-olds should get nine to eleven hours of sleep. And high schoolers should get nine to ten hours of sleep per night.

And it's not just the *quantity* of sleep that matters to your health but the quality as well. An interesting study of young adults showed that slow-wave sleep, which is the most restorative stage of sleep, is important for glucose regulation. When slow-wave sleep is reduced, there is an increased risk of developing type 2 diabetes.

Five Tips for Getting a Good Night's Sleep

Avoid technology in the bedroom. Artificial light from the various technology screens increases alertness and reduces melatonin levels. At least an hour before sleep, turn off the screens.

Practice a regular sleep routine. Start an hour before bed with a relaxing activity, such as reading or taking a bath. Including a regular bedtime and wake-up time as part of your routine are important principles of good sleep hygiene.

Exercise during the day. A sedentary pattern during the day can inhibit nighttime sleepiness. Exercise should not occur within two hours of going to bed.

Stop drinking caffeinated beverages early in the afternoon. The effects of caffeine can last up to eight hours, so if your bedtime is 10:00 p.m., your last cup of coffee should be at 2:00 p.m.

Drink cherry juice, which is rich in melatonin, a natural sleep-inducing chemical. Other common nutritional supplemental remedies include valerian, inositol, lavender, and chamomile, which are easily consumed in herbal teas.

De-stress from the day. Unplug from work and other stressful activities and engage in enjoyable activities before turning in.

Tips for Helping Your Children Get a Better Night's Sleep

Children really need to have a regular bedtime routine. Regular bedtime does not only ensure that a child gets an adequate amount of sleep, but it contributes to a structured environment, which in itself is critical for a child's development. Recent data released by the Princes Trust Youth Index reports that children who lack a daily routine of set bedtimes and mealtimes do worse at school. Moreover, lack of structure contributes to discontentment and lack of confidence in adulthood. The results are far-reaching, impacting a child's future relationships and employability.

I recently evaluated a five-year-old girl (we'll call her Mary) who was brought to the emergency room at midnight for "out-of-control behavior." She had been running through the house, jumping around, and she would not calm down. But this was not unusual for Mary. Her mother stated that Mary usually goes to bed at about 4:00 or 5:00 a.m. and gets up at 2:00 p.m. While she is up all night, Mary is alternately running around the house and watching television. The household, which includes the grandparents, is completely disrupted because of Mary's nocturnal behavior, and Mary's mother complained that her regular pediatrician would not put Mary on a medication for her hyperactivity.

I instructed Mary's mother to gradually wake her earlier in the day and put her to bed earlier each night until she got to a 10:00 p.m. to 6:00 a.m. sleep schedule. Yes, this would take weeks to accomplish, so it would require patience. But a medication would not fix this.

While this is an extreme example, it underscores the point that a bedtime routine is an important strategy for helping children have a healthy night's sleep. Even in their adolescent years, my sons still like me to read to them at night. So my bedtime routine with my children is reading a book, prayer, and then lights out. Two other tips that will help:

- Remove the "screens" from the bedroom. Statistics show that of kids from age eight to eighteen, 71% have a television in their bedroom, and 36% have a computer in their bedroom. Ideally, the bedroom should be free of these devices, but certainly, they should be turned off at least an hour before bedtime.
- Turn off the cell phone during the night. One in ten children report being awakened by text messages during the night (although I'm sure the percentage is higher than that).

So focus this month on getting your optimal amount of sleep every night. One clue that you're getting enough sleep is that you wake up feeling restored without the need for an alarm clock. *Are you up to the challenge?*

Don't forget to continue your

January habit of drinking your optimal amount of water per day (one-half of your weight in ounces of water per day),

February habit of eating seven to nine servings of fruit and vegetables per day,

March habit of replacing refined white foods with whole grains,

April habit of exercising for at least thirty minutes five times per week, and

May habit of detoxifying your system daily.

References

Ahmed, Q, Effects of Common Medications Used for Sleep Disorders, Critical Care Clinics—Volume 24, Issue 3 (July 2008)

Buxton OM, Short and long sleep are positively associated with obesity, diabetes, hypertension, and cardiovascular disease among adults in the United States.——*Soc Sci Med*—01-SEP-2010; 71 (5): 1027-36

Hart, C., Cairns, A., Jelalian, E. Sleep and Obesity in Children and Adolescents. Pediatr Clin N Am 58 (2011) 715-733

Malhotra, R., Desai, A. Healthy Brain Aging: What Has Sleep Got To Do With It?

Clinics in Geriatric Medicine—Volume 26, Issue 1 (February 2010)

Tasali, E., Leproult, R., Ehrmann, D., Van Cauter, E. Slow-wave sleep and the risk of type 2 diabetes in humans. Proc Natl Acad Sci USA, 2008. Jan 22; 105 (3): 1044-9

The association between sleep duration and obesity in older adults. Patel SR—*Int J Obes (Lond)*—01-DEC-2008; 32 (12): 1825-34

The Prince's Trust Youth Index 2012, Released January 2012

Yaggi, HK, Araujo, AB, McKinlay, JB. Sleep duration as a risk factor for the development of type 2 diabetes. Diabetes Care. 2006. March; 29 (3): 657-61

July Challenge

I Will Eat Early, Eat Often, and Stop before It's Too Late!

It's not just what you eat. It's also when you eat. Numerous studies have shown that eating the same number of calories can have a different effect on your weight and health depending on the time of day you consume those calories. So this chapter will arm you with three tips about when to eat to get the most benefit out of your calories.

Tip #1: Eat Early

Do you eat breakfast every day? Or are you like the many people who regularly skip breakfast? The first habit of a healthy day is a nourishing breakfast.

Over the past three decades, obesity rates have been rising rapidly and steadily in both adults and children. It's also been observed that fewer people are eating breakfast. This observation prompted inquiring minds to ask, "Is there a connection?" So researchers did some studies and discovered that there *is* a relationship between eating breakfast and obesity. People who eat breakfast are less likely to be overweight.

One such study was a survey analysis of thirty-five thousand Dutch adolescents, looking at frequency of breakfast skipping, alcohol consumption, and physical activity. The results showed that breakfast skipping had the strongest correlation with being overweight. Another study examining seven hundred ten—to twelve-year-old children showed that consumption of breakfast was inversely related to obesity. Studies also support the notion that the earlier in life a person regularly eats breakfast, the greater the benefits to their long-term health by improved nutritional intake and reduced chance of obesity.

Why is that? (1) Breakfast revs up your metabolism at the start of the day, which helps you burn more calories throughout the day, and (2) people who eat breakfast tend to eat fewer calories during the day than those who skip breakfast.

By the way, parents, chances of a child eating breakfast are significantly increased when a parent is at home during breakfast time. Probably because you're there to say, "Eat your breakfast!" and you're there to prepare breakfast. Another encouraging reason to have your child eat breakfast is that she is likely to continue the habit into adulthood and, therefore, continue receiving the health benefit of breakfast eating.

Does the Type of Breakfast Matter?

Of course it does! Most of the studies looking at breakfast consumption and obesity did not evaluate the type of breakfast eaten. However, if we want to get the most nutritional benefit from breakfast, then we need to choose wisely.

- Choose a high-fiber breakfast. Breakfast is a great time to get a serving of whole grains. Therefore, old-fashioned oatmeal or steel-cut oatmeal is a great breakfast. Avoid instant, quick-cooking, or flavored oatmeal, which are low in fiber and/or high in sugar.
- Add nuts and fruit to your breakfast to further strengthen the nutritional punch. Either a serving of almonds or walnuts added to the oatmeal or a small bowl of fresh fruit on the side is a great way to round out the breakfast.

- Don't be afraid to get unconventional with breakfast. Vegetable medley or beans are a great breakfast choice. My father often eats cucumbers and tomato salad in the morning (usually picked fresh from his garden). You can make a simple bean dip and spread that on your whole grain toast instead of butter.

Not All Cereals Are Created Equal

Beware of boxed breakfast cereals. It's important to read the labels to determine how much sugar and fiber are in those cereals. According to an EWG report of eighty-four breakfast cereals, some breakfast cereals have more sugar than a serving of Hostess Twinkies, which has eighteen grams of sugar. Would you serve Twinkies for breakfast? In fact, only one in four of the cereals reviewed meets the government's guideline of not more than 26% added sugar by weight. Dr. Andrew Weil makes a great point with the following quote:

> When I went to medical school in the 1960s, the consensus view was sugar provided 'empty calories' devoid of vitamins, minerals or fiber. Aside from that, it was not deemed harmful. But 50 years of nutrition research has confirmed that sugar is actually the single most health-destructive component of the standard American diet. The fact that a children's breakfast cereal is 56 percent sugar by weight—and many others are not far behind—should cause national outrage.

In case you're curious, here's the EWG's list of the ten worst cereals *based on percent sugar by weight*:

1. Kellogg's Honey Smacks 55.6%
2. Post Golden Crisp 51.9%
3. Kellogg's Froot Loops Marshmallow 48.3%
4. Quaker Oats Cap'n Crunch's OOPS! All Berries 46.9%
5. Quaker Oats Cap'n Crunch Original 44.4%
6. Quaker Oats Oh!s 44.4%
7. Kellogg's Smorz 43.3%
8. Kellogg's Apple Jacks 42.9%
9. Quaker Oats Cap'n Crunch's Crunch Berries 42.3%
10. Kellogg's Froot Loops Original 41.4%

Tip #2: Eat Often

So which camp do you fall in? The one that eats small meals frequently throughout the day, or the one that has two or three "square meals" per day? If you had to guess, which is better for your health? (What is a square meal anyway?)

Based on the title of this section, you've probably correctly guessed that more frequent meals are the way to go. A study of 4,642 children from age five to six showed that the children who ate five or more meals per day had a lower incidence of obesity than children who ate three or fewer meals per day. A similar trend was found in adolescents. The pattern holds true for adults too. In a cross-sectional study of approximately three thousand men and women, increased meal frequency was associated with a healthier lifestyle. These men and women who ate more frequently tended to eat more carbohydrates and fiber, less fat, protein, and alcohol, and had lower incidence of smoking and higher incidence of physical activity.

What do we mean by frequent eating? Generally, three meals and two or three healthy snacks. This pattern of eating helps keep blood sugar levels steady and keeps you satisfied, thus able to resist binge eating. Healthy snacks are foods that are packed with antioxidants, vitamins, and minerals that keep your metabolism running at a high level. Foods that fit the bill would be vegetables, fruits, nuts, and seeds. For maximum benefit, these snacks need to be organic so that you're not ingesting pesticides and other toxins along with the good stuff.

Tip #3: Stop Before It's Too Late!

Have you noticed the proliferation of twenty-four-hour eating establishments? Lots of fast-food places entice you to grab a late-night meal on your way home. Resist! Your body is simply not designed to eat late at night and process food while you're sleeping. Late eating causes weight gain and leads to all types of digestion problems, especially GERD (gastroesophageal reflux disease). You'll even sleep better when you lie down on a quiet stomach (a stomach that has finished its work of digestion).

A study in mice showed that *when* you eat affects weight gain. Since mice are nocturnal, the researchers fed half of the mice during daytime hours when they would normally sleep, and half the mice were fed during their regular waking hours. The idea was to simulate human eating late at night. Although they ate the exact same number of calories, the mice who ate during the day, their normal sleeping hours, gained more than twice as much weight as the mice who were fed at night.

Researchers believe that this increased weight gain from late-night eating is related to our circadian rhythms. But it has also been observed that people eat larger volume of calories in late-night meals. Therefore, as part of this strategy, you should stop eating about three hours before going to bed.

Tips for Making It Happen

- Stock your pantry with high-fiber and low-sugar breakfast cereals, including some plain whole grains such as oatmeal, millet, and quinoa. I sometimes use a five-grain mix (whole grains of course), and it tastes no different from oatmeal. It takes about five minutes to cook the whole grain oatmeal, compared to thirty seconds in the microwave for instant oatmeal. But it's worth it. You'll save the time in the bathroom later because a high-fiber diet will ensure healthy bowel movement.

- Keep healthy snacks easily accessible. When I put away my groceries, I divide raw vegetables like carrots or broccoli into small ziplock bags. I do the same with nuts and dried fruit. This way, I can just grab a veggie or granola snack from the refrigerator when I'm on the go.

- Get the unhealthy snacks out of your house. It's extremely difficult to resist junk food when you are tired or hungry or stressed out. And don't keep junk food in the house "for the kids." They don't need it any more than you do.

- If you are hungry at bedtime, it's okay to have a small balanced snack (like a piece of fruit dipped in nut butter). That will keep you from waking up from hunger pangs in the middle of the night.

Tip for Kids

I know I don't have to tell you that children are picky. If they have grown accustomed to eating Honey Smacks for breakfast and cookies or chips for their snacks, it will take some creativity and patience to convert to better choices. Make healthy snacks convenient, and make them the only choices except for infrequent occasions. Over time, their grumbling will decrease, and they won't remember the "old way."

It's a three-part challenge for the month of July, but you can handle it. Remember, you are building habits that will result in optimal health for the rest of your life.

FAQs

How often can I have bacon and eggs?

Bacon is one of the worst foods you can eat because it is extremely high in saturated fat. It really is a strip of meat sandwiched in animal fat. Bacon cannot be considered part of a healthy breakfast. I recommend that you omit it completely. Eggs should be eaten sparingly, no more than twice per week.

I'm never hungry at breakfast time. What should I do?

If you normally have a low appetite in the morning, that will probably be corrected by not eating within three to four hours of bedtime. But if you still feel unmotivated to eat breakfast, just keep it light. Even simply eating a piece of fruit will break the fast and start your metabolism. You can work your way up to a heartier breakfast. Just like anything else, breakfast eating is a habit that may take time get used to.

I work at night. How does this eating schedule affect me?

If you consistently work at night and sleep during the day, just reverse the recommendations to fit your schedule. If you work varying shifts (like I have in the past), it's more of a challenge. The principle is the same: regular meals during your waking hours with power-packed snacks.

Don't forget to continue your

January habit of drinking your optimal amount of water per day (one-half of your weight in ounces of water per day),

February habit of eating seven to nine servings of fruit and vegetables per day,

March habit of replacing refined white foods with whole grains,

April habit of exercising for at least thirty minutes five times per week,

May habit of detoxifying your system daily, and

June habit of sleeping for seven to eight hours each night.

References

Croezen S. Skipping breakfast, alcohol consumption and physical inactivity as risk factors for overweight and obesity in adolescents: results of the E-MOVO project.—*Eur J Clin Nutr*—01-MAR-2009; 63 (3): 405-12

EWG News Release, December 7, 2012 Kids' Cereals Pack More Sugar Than Twinkies and Cookies

Meal patterns and childhood obesity.—Patro B—*Curr Opin Clin Nutr Metab Care*—01-MAY-2010; 13 (3): 300-4

Merten, M., Williams, A., Shriver, L. Breakfast Consumption in Adolescence and Young Adulthood: Parental presence, community context and obesity.

Panagiotakos D. Breakfast cereal is associated with a lower prevalence of obesity among 10-12-year-old children: the PANACEA study.—*Nutr Metab Cardiovasc Dis*—01-NOV-2008; 18 (9): 606-12

September 3, 2009, *1:24 pm,* Late Night Eating Linked to Weight Gain *By TARA PARKER-POPE New York Times. http://well.blogs. nytimes.com/2009/09/03/late-night-eating-linked-to-weight-gain/*

Toschke, A. Meal Frequency, breakfast consumption and childhood obesity. Int J Pediatr Obes. 01-Jan-2009; 4 (4): 242-8

August Challenge

I Will Protect My Heart and Brain by Enriching My Diet with Omega-3 Fatty Acid Power!

Of the three macronutrients—protein, carbohydrates, and fat—we tend to think of fat as a bad actor. We all want to get rid of fat and often hear the message that fat needs to be avoided in the diet. But not all fat is created equally. Saturated fats and trans fats are major contributors to heart disease, but some types of fat support heart health, and those include the omega-3 fatty acids.

You mean, fats can be good for you? The right kinds of fat are more than good—they're essential. Omega-3 fatty acids are called essential because the body doesn't manufacture them, and so they have to be acquired in food sources. Omega-3 fatty acids are polyunsaturated fatty acids found in marine and plant sources. Marine sources provide DHA (docosahexaenoic acid) and EPA (eicosapentaenoic acid); plant sources mostly provide ALA (alpha-linolenic acid).

The Benefits of Omega-3 Fatty Acids

Omega-3 fatty acids improve cardiovascular risk factors by (1) antiplatelet activity (platelets cause clotting of the blood and, therefore, can lead to poor circulation), (2) triglyceride reduction (of course, high triglycerides are a risk factor for cardiovascular disease), (3) increased HDL cholesterol (the good cholesterol, as it's called because it prevents atherosclerosis).

Omega-3 fatty acids reduce cardiovascular mortality. Intake of DHA and EPA is associated with decreased risk of cardiovascular events. A study called the Diet and Reinfarction Trial found a 29% reduction in two-year all-cause mortality in recovered myocardial infarction (heart attack) patients who ate two servings of fatty fish per week. Another study, entitled the GISSSO-Prevenzione Study, found that one gram per day of fish oil reduced overall risk of mortality by 20%, cardiovascular disease mortality by 30%, and sudden death by 47%. A study in Japan showed that a combination of EPA treatment and statin drug (a common cholesterol drug) reduced major coronary events by 19% and unstable angina incidence by 28% compared to the statin drug alone.

Omega-3 fatty acids improve inflammatory conditions. Omega-3 fatty acids are thought to be beneficial in some inflammatory-related diseases by displacing omega-6 fatty acids, including arachidonic acid, in the cell membrane. This reduces the creation of metabolic end products, including prostaglandins, thromboxanes, and leukotrienes.

Omega-3 fatty acids are also a great brain-health nutrient. Our brains are 60% fat, and therefore, healthy fats are needed to support the structure and function of the brain. Omega-3 fatty acids play a central role in the development and function of the central nervous system by contributing to the structure of and communication between brain cells. Decreased DHA has been shown to impair production of nerve cells, metabolism of neurotransmitters (chemical messengers between nerve cells), learning, and vision. Also, by lowering inflammation, omega-3s protect against neurological (such as Alzheimer's) and psychological (such as depression) conditions.

Omega-3 fatty acids help psychiatric disorders. An interesting study was done to examine anxiety in medical students (about the most anxious people you can find). In this small questionnaire study of sixty-eight healthy young medical students, anxiety levels were found to be 20% lower in those who were taking fish oil supplements compared to those taking a placebo. Studies have also connected low omega-3 levels to stress, depression, and schizophrenia.

In his book, *The Brain Diet*, Dr. Alan Logan states, "Dietary and supplemental omega-3 fatty acids may be the most significant brain insurance policy you can purchase."

Where Are Good sources of Omega-3 Fatty Acids?

- Fatty fish, such as salmon and tuna. When eating salmon, always choose wild-caught as opposed to farm-raised salmon. Wild-caught salmon is much healthier because, due to its diet of mainly algae, it has a much-higher content of DHA, and lower content of arachidonic acid (a pro-inflammatory chemical).
- Nuts and seeds. Walnuts are an excellent plant source of omega-3s. Seeds such as pumpkin seeds, flax seeds, and chia seeds are also great sources. Flax seeds need to be ground up for our bodies to absorb their nutrients.
- Omega-3 fatty acid supplements, which will be further discussed in chapter 12.

Tips for Incorporating Sources of Omega-3 Fatty Acids Daily into Your Diet

Use nuts and seeds as snacks. I like to make baggies of walnuts and dried fruit to grab quickly when I'm on the run or to pack for snacking at work.

Sprinkle ground flax seeds or chia seeds into your morning oatmeal or into your homemade frozen smoothie.

Eat a serving of fatty fish twice per week.

What You Can Expect from *This One Change*

Decreased aches and pains. Because of their anti-inflammatory effect, omega-3 fatty acids can provide relief for painful inflammatory conditions that affect the joints, muscles, and other organs of the body.

Improved mood. Omega-3 fatty acids have been shown to reduce anxiety, depression, or other mood disorders.

Improved mental clarity. By strengthening brain structure and function, omega-3 fatty acids improve cognitive performance.

Tip for Kids

While all of us need some fat in our diet, babies and young toddlers have the largest need. In fact, nature's perfect baby food, which is breast milk, is 50% fat by calories. As mentioned above, DHA is a critical omega-3 fatty acid for brain health because of its role in the structure and communication of brain cells. Breast milk (unlike cow's milk) contains DHA. However, you should know that the level of DHA in breast milk varies widely based on maternal intake. Therefore, if you're pregnant, be sure to fortify your diet with foods packed with omega-3 (with the exception of fish and supplements that are tainted with mercury).

A Surprising Source of Omega-3 Power

Here's a little known secret: a great source of omega-3 fatty acids can be found in chia seeds. In fact, chia seeds are the most abundant plant source of omega-3. A great property of these seeds is that you can soak them in water for fifteen minutes, and they will form a gel that you can use to create a pudding or gelatin dessert. And chia seeds have the added benefit of being a great source of fiber, calcium, antioxidants, protein, and other nutrients. A lot of power in a tiny package!

Don't forget to continue your

January habit of drinking your optimal amount of water per day (one-half of your weight in ounces of water per day),

February habit of eating seven to nine servings of fruit and vegetables per day,

March habit of replacing refined white foods with whole grains,

April habit of exercising for at least thirty minutes five times per week,

May habit of detoxifying your system daily,

June habit of sleeping for seven to eight hours each night, and

July habit of eating early, eating often, and stopping before it's too late.

References

Chilton, F. & Tucker, L. (2006). *Inflammation Nation*. New York, NY: Fireside.

Logan, A. *The Brain Diet*. (2006). Nashville, TN, Cumberland House Publishing. 4

Katcher, H., Hill, A., Lanford, J., Yoo, J., Kris-Etherton, P. Lifestyle Approaches and Dietary Strategies to Lower LDL-Cholesterol and Triglycerides and Raise HDL-Cholesterol. *Endocrinology and Metabolism Clinics*—Volume 38, Issue 1 (March 2009)

Kiecolt-Glaser JK, Belury MA, Andridge R, et al. Omega3 supplementation lowers inflammation and anxiety in medical students: a randomized controlled trial. *Brain, Behavior, and Immunity*. 2011.

White, B. Dietary Fatty Acids. American Family Physician—Volume 80, Issue 4 (August 2009

SEPTEMBER CHALLENGE

My Family Will Share a Home-Cooked Meal Together at Least Five Times Each Week

September is the time of the year when summer is coming to an end and the kids are back in school; most of us are settling back into a daily routine. Let me encourage you to make family meals part of your daily routine. If not every day, at least five times per week should be doable for most families.

Fewer families are sharing meals together. We can imagine why. The pace of life has substantially increased in recent years. Economic pressures often force parents to work longer hours and farther from home, adding commute time to an already long day. Work is often following parents home as well. Children are involved in many extracurricular activities, sometimes requiring them to participate in long practice sessions several nights per week, if not every night. And of course, homework needs to be done once the children make it home. Therefore, the family dinner is becoming crowded out. This is a great loss and is having detrimental health effects on our children and us adults alike.

Studies show that children who eat with their families more often are less likely to be overweight. Why is that? Most likely because the home-prepared meals that the children are eating are more healthy than store-bought foods. And at the table, the parent is able to influence the child's attitudes toward healthful diets. But the rewards extend far beyond a healthy weight. Family meals affect a child's emotional, psychological, and social health as well.

One of the most comprehensive studies on this topic has been produced by the National Center on Addiction and Substance Abuse at Columbia University (CASA), who conducted a survey of 1,037 teenagers from age twelve to seventeen (546 males, 491 females) and 528 parents of these teens via the Internet. According to their 2011 report,

> Our surveys have consistently found a relationship between children having frequent dinners with their parents and a decreased risk of their smoking, drinking or using other drugs, and that parental engagement fostered around the dinner table is one of the most potent tools to help parents raise healthy, drug-free children. Simply put: frequent family dinners make a difference.

Here is a partial list of research-proven benefits that children experience from frequent family meals:

- Formation of healthy eating habits in the future
- Decreased future substance use and eating disorders
- Improved emotional well-being in adolescents
- Increased intake of vegetables
- Increased intake of vitamins and minerals

It probably comes as no surprise to you that sharing meals together as a family produces healthy, emotionally balanced children. When we are able to gather around the table with our loved ones, we can recover from the stresses of the day in an atmosphere of acceptance and security. The family table is also an ideal environment to pass on parental values both in words and, more important, modeling. A recent study from the Prince's Trust Youth Index found that regular mealtimes contribute to a child's attainment of academic success, resiliency, and social skills.

Given the importance of this habit, here are some tips for making it work:

- Make the family table a media-free zone. That is, turn off the television and prohibit cell phones and computers at the table. That will help everyone at the table give their attention to one another.
- Tame time-stealers to protect the family meal hour. You may have to be ruthless about clearing some activities from your schedule and that of the kids to ensure an opportunity to gather together for a family meal at least five times per week.
- Always have plenty of fruits and vegetables on the table. Kids are more likely to eat the healthy options when they are right in front of them.
- Plan ahead and use quick cooking methods, such as sautéing and broiling, for healthy and quickly prepared meals.

Helping Children Value Family Meals

You may think your children outgrow the need or desire for family time as they get older. Sure, teenagers highly value their friends and opportunities for constant communication with them through texting and social media. But at any age, they still need, and usually want, to spend time with their parents and siblings. The research study by CASA, released in 2011, bears this out:

This year's study again demonstrates that the magic that happens at family dinners isn't the food on the table, but the conversations and family engagement around the table. When asked about the best part of family dinners, the most frequent answer from teens is the sharing, talking and interacting with family members; the second most frequent answer is sitting down or being together. Add in similar responses such as spending time with particular family members or laughing and telling jokes, and the result is that three-quarters of teens who report having dinner with their family at least once a week find the interaction and being together to be the best part of family dinners.

For great ideas about family dinners, visit www.CASAFamilyDay.org.

Don't forget to continue your

January habit of drinking your optimal amount of water per day (one-half of your weight in ounces of water per day),

February habit of eating seven to nine servings of fruit and vegetables per day,

March habit of replacing refined white foods with whole grains,

April habit of exercising for at least thirty minutes five times per week,

May habit of detoxifying your system daily,

June habit of sleeping for seven to eight hours each night,

July habit of eating early, eating often, and stopping before it's too late, and

August habit of increasing omega-3 fatty acids in your diet.

References

Are family meal patterns associated with overall diet quality during the transition from early to middle adolescence?—Burgess-Champoux TL—*J Nutr Educ Behav*—01-MAR-2009; 41 (2): 79-86

Family meals and adolescents: what have we learned from Project EAT (Eating Among Teens)?—Neumark-Sztainer D—*Public Health Nutr*—01-JUL-2010; 13 (7): 1113-21

The Prince's Trust Youth Index 2012, Released January 2012

The Importance of Family Dinners, VII; Sept 2011. National Center on Addiction and Substance Abuse at Columbia University. http://www.casacolumbia.org/upload/2011/2011922familydinnersVII.pdf

OCTOBER CHALLENGE

I Will Restrict My Media Diet

Looking for a way to

- lose weight?
- reduce your cravings for unhealthy foods?
- reduce your stress levels?
- reduce your children's chances of using alcohol, tobacco, and illicit drugs?
- reduce your children's chances of initiating sex at an early age?
- improve your children's academic performance?

Of course you are. That's why you are reading this book. Is there one healthy habit that can achieve all these things? Of course there is, or I wouldn't have asked the question. Changing our media diet is a key strategy to accomplishing these goals!

What Is Our Current Media Diet?

Just like the average calorie intake of Americans has increased over the past few decades, so has our media consumption. It could only be expected with the myriad of media options we now have. Television viewing no longer requires a television set now that we can view television programming on our computers, smart phones, and portable DVDs (including in our cars). And we now have all those same options to surf the Internet and keep current on social media sites.

The average American watches about 151 hours of television per month, which is almost 40 hours per week, the equivalent of a full-time job! That's almost 6 hours per day. By the time you add in cell phone use, computers, and other devices, American adults are up to about 8 hours per day. That's followed closely behind by our children. On average, children and teens are spending 7 hours per day with media.

So What's the Problem?

This huge appetite for media is wreaking havoc on our health. Let's look at how:

- Media affects our weight. Media consumption is a sedentary activity. Well, not always. More and more we're seeing people show up to the emergency rooms with broken limbs because of trying to engage in their media while walking (falling off curbs, walking into the street with oncoming traffic, etc.). Anyway, you know that a sedentary lifestyle is a strong contributor to weight gain. In a recent study, it was found that children who consume media for more than two hours daily *and* who have less daily physical activity than recommended were three to four times more likely to be overweight.
- Media has another powerful way of helping us put on the pounds, and that's through advertising. Several very intriguing studies have looked at the food advertising during prime time and during Saturday morning kids' programming. Turns out that a two-thousand-calorie diet consisting of purely advertised foods on prime time television would give you *twenty-five times* the recommended

servings of sugar, *twenty times* the recommended servings of fat, and *less than half* the recommended servings of fruits, vegetables, and dairy per day. The vast majority of food promoted on television also contains low-quality grains (i.e., mostly refined, low-fiber grains) and a deficiency of many important minerals and vitamins, such as calcium, magnesium, and vitamin E.

- Media causes behavior changes in children; of course, the media loves to deny this and regularly refutes these findings. But numerous studies show the powerful effect of media on the behavior of children:

  - More than two thousand scientific studies and reviews show that significant exposure to media violence increases aggressive behavior, desensitizes children to violence, and frightens them into believing that the world is more dangerous than it actually is.
  - Research is finding that the highly sexualized content of media programming (usually neglecting to mention any negative consequences) may contribute to early sexual intercourse among teens.
  - Smoking and drinking alcohol are frequently shown in the media, often in a glamorized light. A recent meta-analysis estimated that "44% of all smoking initiation among children and young teenagers could be attributed to viewing smoking in movies." Research is also showing that alcohol advertising is very effective in convincing teens to drink.

- Media also affects attention and school performance. An interesting study looked at the effects of certain types of programming on children's executive function—that is, their ability to plan, organize, and control their behavior.

The study showed that merely nine minutes of watching a fast-paced cartoon resulted in a significantly worse performance on executive-functioning tasks compared to watching an educational cartoon or drawing.

These results should not surprise us, although I hope it disturbs us. I believe that there are many other negative effects to this overconsumption of media that cannot be as easily quantified. For example, what is happening to our social interaction? It is becoming more and more acceptable to text at the dining table. At a time when family members should be interacting with one another, they are often using a significant proportion of their attention engaged in "conversations" with people who are miles away. Shouldn't we value one another more than that?

Several years ago, I was on a school trip with my younger son as a parent chaperone. As the children were engaging in a hands-on activity, I noticed one of the parents completely engaged with his smart phone the entire time. He never looked at his child's activity or engaged in it with him. And this is becoming more common. Children are having a harder time getting their parents' attention and are often left to entertain themselves as their parents attend to their cell phones, computers, or televisions. Although this is not completely new, it's certainly more prevalent than it was years ago. And it has caused me to adopt a term that my sister Gloria coined, "the new child abuse" because children are sometimes engaging in dangerous behavior (e.g., exploring electrical sockets, running out into the street) right under the noses of their distracted parents.

But I digress. Changing our media diet, by reducing consumption, is an important step to restoring our physical, mental, emotional, and social health. So what should our media diet be?

○ For kids less than two, the American Academy of Pediatrics recommends no screen time. Children in this age group learn much more effectively by interacting with a person rather than a screen.

○ For kids older than two, no more than two hours of good-quality programming per day.

○ For adults, there is no official recommendation, but I suggest that you be the role model by limiting your own screen time, and spend much more of that time being active and interacting with live people.

What You Can Expect from *This One Change*

- *Weight loss.* By replacing screen time with more physical activity, you will be on your way to achieve a healthy weight.
- *Improved mood.* Physical activity releases hormones that improve our mood
- *Better school performance and reading ability.*

Getting Outdoors

An important alternative to being in front of the screen is spending more time outdoors. In his book *Last Child in the Woods*, Richard Louv makes a strong case for the positive impact of the natural environment on the physical and psychological health of children.

He states, "More time in nature—combined with less television and more stimulating play and educational settings—may go a long way toward reducing attention deficits in children, and, just as important, increasing their joy in life."

Suggestions to Make It Happen

- Find fun alternatives to screen time. Children still enjoy board games and outdoor play as long as they have others to enjoy these activities with.
- Accept the challenge to unplug for a period of time. Family Life Today is one of several organizations that promote TV-free week every year. See how creative your family can be when you give up the entertainment options of the television and computer.
- Allow children to be bored. Sometimes, they'll complain that they have nothing to do. This is a great time for them to get creative in developing ways to entertain themselves. In fact, I believe children and adults need more quiet time to get in touch with our spirits and for personal development and growth.
- Keep children's bedrooms television-free (more than 70% of teens have a television in their rooms). This can cut down on total television viewing time, but more importantly, it can reduce viewing of late-night television shows that tend to have increased violence and sexual content.
- Turn the television off at mealtimes so that the dinner table can be a place of interaction between family members. When children are relaxed around the table with their parents' attention, they may divulge some of their concerns and challenges.

Don't forget to continue your

January habit of drinking your optimal amount of water per day (one-half of your weight in ounces of water per day),

February habit of eating seven to nine servings of fruit and vegetables per day,

March habit of replacing refined white foods with whole grains,

April habit of exercising for at least thirty minutes five times per week,

May habit of detoxifying your system daily,

June habit of sleeping for seven to eight hours each night,

July habit of eating early, eating often, and stopping before it's too late,

August habit of increasing omega-3 fatty acids in your diet, and

September habit of sharing a home-cooked meal with your family at least five times per week.

References

Americans spend eight hours a day on screens Mar 27 01:18 PM US/Eastern http://www.breitbart.com/article.php?id=CNG.9 2e661444313b232e8931de00c29c73b.431

Batada, A., Seitz, M., Wootan, M., Story, M. Nine out of 10 Food Advertisements Shown During Saturday Morning Children's Television Programming Are for Foods High in Fat, Sodium, or Added Sugars, or Low in Nutrients. *Journal of the American Dietetic Association*—Volume 108, Issue 4 (April 2008)

Laurson, K., Eisenmann, J., Welk, G., Wickel, E., Gentile, D., Walsh, D Combined Influence Of Physical Activity And Screen Time Recommendations On Childhood Overweight. *Journal of Pediatrics*—Volume 153, Issue 2 (August 2008)

Lillard, A., Peterson, J. The immediate impact of different types of television on young children's executive function. *Pediatrics.* 2011; 128: 644-649

Louv, Richard (2008) Last Child in the Woods: Saving Our Children From Nature-Deficit Disorder. Algonquin Books.

Mink, M; Evans, A. Phd; Moore, C; Calderon, K., Deger, S. Nutritional Imbalance Endorsed By Televised Food Advertisements, *Journal Of The American Dietetic Association*—Volume 110, Issue 6 (June 2010)

Rettew, David. In this Issue/Abstract Thinking: Media and Children's Mental Health. *Journal of the American Academy of Child and Adolescent Psychiatry*—Volume 47, Issue 5 (May 2008)

TV viewing at 'all-time high,' Nielsen says. February 24, 2009 By Taylor Gandossy CNN http://articles.cnn.com/2009-02-24/ entertainment/us.video.nielsen_1_nielsen-company-nielsen-spokesman-gary-holmes-watching?_s=PM:SHOWBIZ

November Challenge

I Will Start Practicing Stress-Reducing Strategies Every Day

When we hear the word *stress*, we often think of it as a psychological issue. We do not usually think about stress as having physical effects on our bodies. Yet our minds and bodies are intimately linked together, and so it should be no surprise that stress affects our bodies. In fact, there is a field of study called psychoneuroimmunology, which studies the relationships between stress and physical health. Stress activates a host of chemical messengers in our bodies that contribute to dysfunction of different body systems, such as our cardiovascular and immune systems.

Webster's dictionary describes *stress* as "a physical, chemical, or emotional factor that causes bodily or mental tension." Many of these "factors" are things that we cannot control. Therefore, reducing stress is often not possible. For example, when we find ourselves having to care for a disabled family member or when we experience a job loss, we cannot reduce the stress of those situations. However, we can protect our bodies and minds from being damaged by stress by practicing stress-reducing strategies.

How Does Stress Affect My Health?

About 80% of diseases are stress related! Life stress activates a cascade effect in the brain that causes the body to release catecholamines and cortisol, which are chemicals and hormones that have a variety of effects in the body. Let's look at the most well-described effects of stress:

Stress affects the cardiovascular system by

- increasing blood pressure,
- increasing blood thickness (making it more prone to clot),
- increasing inflammation,
- increasing production and release of triglycerides from the liver, and
- increasing LDL (bad cholesterol).

The ultimate effects of all these changes are increased incidence of coronary artery disease, chronic hypertension, and heart attacks.

Stress impairs the immune system. It has been observed that high stress populations experience increased rates of infections. We now know that stress suppresses immunity, which leads to greater susceptibility to infections. By impairing the immune system, chronic stress also delays wound healing, impairs response to vaccinations, and leads to faster progression of diseases. On the other hand, stress enhances the inflammatory components of the immune system, which exacerbates inflammatory conditions such as asthma, allergies, and autoimmune diseases.

Stress impairs the gastrointestinal system. Have you ever been under stress and felt "knots" in your stomach? Developed diarrhea? Lost your appetite? Many people have these types of reactions to stress because the brain and gut are intimately connected.

Therefore, chronic stress often leads to digestive dysfunction and chronic abdominal pain. Common GI diseases associated with stress include irritable bowel syndrome, peptic ulcers (infectious causes notwithstanding), and even ulcerative colitis.

Stress is also associated with obesity. A study of Swedish families found that children in a stressful family situation had a significantly higher incidence of obesity compared to those in low-stress family environments.

So given how extensively stress affects so many aspects of our bodies' functioning, we can see why stress is a key underlying contributor to up to 80% of chronic diseases. Therefore, we must learn stress-reducing strategies if we are going to experience incredible health.

Effective Stress-Reducing Strategies

- *Exercise.* Exercise reduces stress hormone release, and the effects last for hours after exercise is finished. Exercise also makes you feel good by causing the release of endorphins (feel-good chemicals) in the brain. But since the stress-reduction benefit of exercise is temporary, it's only an effective tool if done regularly. Remember to make it fun!
- *Choose optimism.* Are people born optimists or pessimists? Some people think so. But even if you have a tendency to see the glass as half empty, you can choose optimism. As shown in a study by researcher Giltay, people who reported high levels of optimism had a 55% lower risk of death from all causes and a 23% lower risk of cardiovascular death.
- *Get connected.* Connection with family members, friends, and community groups have all been shown to decrease life stress. For example, a thirty-five-year prospective study showed that a warm relationship with parents in early life carried a significantly decreased risk of heart disease,

cancer, and all-cause mortality in adulthood. A similar fifty-year study of medical students also found that closeness to parents reduced the likelihood of cancer, heart disease, suicide, and interpersonal difficulties. Moreover, positive health effects were shown with warm marital relationships. Connection with others is thought to positively impact physical health through reduction of stress hormones and through improvement of immune function. On the other hand, social isolation is a significant risk factor for coronary artery disease, cancer, and all-cause mortality. Therefore, maintaining relationships with family and friends and participating in support groups are important to your health.

- *Meditate.* Meditation has been shown to reduce stress-hormone levels and to decrease the "fight or flight" response that the body assumes when you're stressed out. To meditate simply means to focus your thoughts on something or to reflect on something. It means to "think on these things." Meditation is a tool that allows you to draw upon your inner resources to bring clarity and calmness to difficult situations. Meditation works best when it is a daily practice. The best-selling book of all time, the Bible, strongly encourages us to meditate. An abundance of research has looked at the effects of meditation on physical illness and has found that the practice of meditation has beneficial effects in the treatment of the following disorders:

  - tension
  - headaches
  - psoriasis
  - blood pressure
  - serum cholesterol
  - smoking cessation

- ° alcohol abuse
- ° carotid atherosclerosis
- ° coronary artery disease
- ° longevity and cognitive function in the elderly
- ° psychiatric disorders
- ° excessive worry
- ° use of medical care
- ° chronic pain

Meditation is undoubtedly a powerful stress-reducing tool.

Helping Children Cope with Stress

Children face stress on a daily basis just as adults do. An important tool that children can develop to effectively deal with stressful situations is the characteristic of resilience. In his book *Please Don't Label My Child,* psychiatrist Scott Shannon defines *resilience* as "the ability to bounce back in the face of adversity" and offers the following tips for building resilience into your child:

- Encourage your child to take risks to reach her goals.
- Respect your child's problem-solving skills.
- Encourage your child to find support.
- Encourage your child to volunteer and help others.
- Encourage your child to openly express his needs, desires, and opinions.
- Encourage your child to practice self-examination and reflection.

Don't forget to continue your

January habit of drinking your optimal amount of water per day (one-half of your weight in ounces of water per day),

February habit of eating seven to nine servings of fruit and vegetables per day,

March habit of replacing refined white foods with whole grains,

April habit of exercising for at least thirty minutes five times per week,

May habit of detoxifying your system daily,

June habit of sleeping for seven to eight hours each night,

July habit of eating early, eating often, and stopping before it's too late,

August habit of increasing omega-3 fatty acids in your diet,

September habit of sharing a home-cooked meal with your family at least five times per week, and

October habit of reducing your media diet.

References

Cacioppo JT. Social neuroscience: autonomic, neuroendocrine, and immune response to stress. *Psychophysiology*. 1994; 31: 113-128

Fortney, L. and Taylor, M. Meditation in Medical Practice: A Review of the Evidence and Practice Primary Care: Clinics in Office Practice—Volume 37, Issue 1 (March 2010)

Giltay EJ, Geleijnse JM, Zitman FG, Hoekstra T, Schouten EG. Dispositional optimism and all-cause and cardiovascular mortality in a prospective cohort of elderly dutch men and women. Arch Gen Psychiatry. 2004 Nov; 61 (11): 1126-35.

Koch, F., Sepa, A., Ludvigsson, J. Psychological Stress and Obesity. The Journal of Pediatrics. December 2008.

Larzelere, M., Jones, G. Stress and Health. Prim Care Clin Office Pract 35 (2008) 839-856.

Marshall, G. The adverse effects of psychological stress on immunoregulatory balance: applications to human inflammatory diseases. *Immunol Allergy Clin N Am* 31 (2011) 133-140.

Russek LG, King SH, Russek SJ, Russek HI. The Harvard Mastery of Stress Study 35-year follow-up: prognostic significance of patterns of psychophysiological arousal and adaptation. *Psychosom Med.* 1990; 52 (3): 271-85.

Shannon, Scott. Please Don't Label My Child (2007) New York, NY, Rodale Publishing Thomas CB, Duszynski KR. Closeness to parents and the family constellation in a prospective study of five disease states: suicide, mental illness, malignant tumor, hypertension and coronary artery disease. *Johns Hopkins Medical Journal.* 1974; 134: 251.

DECEMBER CHALLENGE

I Will Optimize My Daily Diet with the Proper Supplements

Congratulations for making it this far! The habit you'll develop in this chapter is what I call the icing on the cake. I purposely left it for last because this habit is powerful only in conjunction with a healthy diet and lifestyle.

Most people in America take some combination of nutritional supplements, and many people are very confused as to what they should take. Have you ever walked into a nutritional shop and felt overwhelmed with the options? I have. There are individual herbs, herbal formulations, homeopathic formulations, vitamin-and-mineral combinations, enzyme powders, and an assortment of miscellaneous substances. Many of these products claim to help with whatever ails you: sleep aids, digestion aids, energy potions, mood lifters, etc. How can you possibly know what to take? And do we really need supplements at all, or does a healthy diet provide all the nutrition that we need?

I find that people make three common mistakes with supplements:

1. Trying out whatever supplements they find labeled for their particular health concern using a "grab bag" approach,

2. Switching from one product to another based on the latest news release in an attempt to feel better overall, and
3. Just taking a single megavitamin in hopes of covering everything with one super pill.

When I first started studying supplementation, I was overwhelmed and confused. After months of study, I came to the conclusion that, yes, we do need to supplement our diets for maximal health. The good news is that supplementation needs are very simple for the average person. While supplementation can get complex for people with specific disorders, what follows is my recommended three supplements that I believe everyone can benefit from, even with a healthy diet.

Three Reasons We Need Supplements

- Our food supply is woefully lacking in vitamin-and-mineral content. Consider this: many of our fruits, vegetables, and grains have only a fraction of the nutrients they had half a century ago. This is because of farming practices that have led to soil depletion.
- The most recent Cancer Trends Progress Report published by the National Cancer Institute recommends that we eat up to thirteen servings of fresh fruits and vegetables per day. Most Americans do not come close to that. Hopefully, now that you have read this book, *you* are eating at least seven servings daily.
- Most Americans are not eating close to the recommended levels of whole grains daily, which are a powerful source of B vitamins and important minerals.

That being said, I recommend the following three supplements:

1. Whole food daily supplements
2. Vitamin D
3. Omega-3 fatty acids

Let's look at each one individually.

Whole Food Supplements

Whole food supplements are dehydrated, cold-processed plant foods in a powder that provide concentrated vitamins and minerals in their whole state. That's important because our bodies are designed to process nutrients from food, not to process fractionated chemicals. For example, an apple contains hundreds, if not thousands, of compounds that work synergistically to nourish our bodies. But a multivitamin incorporates just a few of those nutrients, such as ascorbate and zinc.

Whole food supplements come in a variety of formulations. Some focus on green vegetables and grasses, whereas others are combinations of fruits and vegetables. The most important factor to consider is the manufacturing process. The supplement you take should be created from the whole fruit or vegetable, which includes the skins, and should be created under a low-heat process in order to preserve the nutrients. Also, your supplement should not contain artificial colors, flavors, or sweeteners.

Whole food supplements are very different from multivitamins. I consider whole food supplements to be superior to multivitamins as a daily supplement for the following reasons:

- Our bodies only absorb about a small fraction of synthetic vitamins. That bright yellow urine that you see after you've taken a vitamin is the majority of your hard-earned money in the toilet.
- The fractionated chemicals that compose typical vitamins are often ineffective. Studies have consistently failed to show increased longevity or reduction of disease risk from use of multivitamins. As stated by Dr. Timothy O'Shea:

> Vitamins cannot be isolated from their complexes and still perform their specific life functions within the cells. When isolated into artificial commercial forms, like ascorbic acid, these purified synthetics act as drugs in the body. They are no longer vitamins, and to call them such is inaccurate.

- Megadoses of vitamins can be toxic. For example, several recent large studies indicate that people with high levels of vitamin A in their blood have a greater risk for osteoporosis. Another study has linked excessive vitamin A with lung cancer.

High doses of specific vitamins have been shown to significantly benefit certain conditions, and therefore, I am not suggesting that vitamins are not helpful in particular cases. However, for overall daily supplementation, a whole food supplement provides much richer nourishment for the body than a multivitamin.

Vitamin D

Vitamin D deficiency has risen to epidemic levels. It is estimated that between 25% and 57% of Americans are deficient in vitamin D, which refers to a vitamin D level of less than 20 ng/ml. While we call it a vitamin, it's actually a hormone that is produced in the body. The major source of vitamin D is through exposure to sunlight. For example, just ten to fifteen minutes of sunlight exposure can generate 10,000 to 20,000 IU of vitamin D. (People with darker skin may require five to ten times that length of time for the same resulting levels.) Sufficient vitamin D is difficult to obtain from foods. Good sources are fatty fish, such as salmon, mackerel, or sardines. Cod liver oil is a good source. Vitamin D can also be obtained from fortified foods, such as cereals.

Most people associate vitamin D with bone health because, historically, vitamin D deficiency has been associated with rickets, or brittle bone disease. We now know that vitamin D deficiency is associated with a multitude of diseases other than bone disease.

- Vitamin D deficiency is associated with greater cancer risk. Numerous studies have shown a correlation between low vitamin D levels and increased incidence of cancer, while clinical trials have also shown reduced risk by vitamin D3 supplementation.
- Vitamin D has been shown to be an effective treatment for psoriasis.
- Vitamin D supplementation reduces incidence of autoimmune diseases, specifically multiple sclerosis and type 1 diabetes (when taken during infancy). Vitamin D deficiency in mothers is also associated with increased incidence of asthma and wheezing disorders in their children.
- Vitamin D enhances the immune response and provides protection against upper respiratory infections, influenza, and middle ear infections.
- Vitamin D deficiency also affects the cardiovascular system. Deficiency of vitamin D increases the risk for heart attack, hypertension, peripheral vascular disease, metabolic syndrome, coronary artery disease, and heart failure.

So you can see that vitamin D is essential for optimal functioning of the entire body, not just our bones.

So how much vitamin D should you take? Infants, especially breast-fed infants, should take 400 IU of vitamin D per day. Children over age one may take 400 to 1,000 IU of vitamin D per day. Adults should take 2,000 IU of vitamin D per day. The best form of vitamin D supplementation is vitamin D3.

Omega-3 Fatty Acids

In the chapter on omega-3 power, I listed the numerous health benefits of getting adequate omega-3 levels. To briefly recap, omega-3 fatty acids are essential for cardiovascular and brain health. They help protect against inflammatory diseases, psychiatric disorders, neurologic diseases, and cardiovascular diseases. Therefore, I recommend daily supplementation with omega-3 fatty acid that contains both DHA and EPA.

Tips for Making It Happen

Make sure to use high-quality supplements. Many companies try to compete with one another by selling inexpensive supplements, but some of these may be inferior in quality. Look for the "USP verified" (United States Pharmacopeia) label. This indicates that (1) the listed ingredients are present in the product and in the amounts indicated, (2) the product does not contain harmful levels of specified contaminants, (3) the product was made using good manufacturing practices (GMP), and (4) the supplement will break down and release its contents into the body. NSF is a similar quality label that you should look for. Another good resource is ConsumerLab.com for investigating the quality of a nutritional supplement.

For omega-3 supplementation, I recommend Nordic Naturals products. They are high quality and have a variety of formulations that are easy for children to use.

For whole food supplementation, I use, and am a distributor for Juice Plus+, the most thoroughly researched nutritional supplement in the market. It is a high-quality combination of fruits and vegetables and also has a good formulation for kids.

Make your nutritional supplements easy for you to remember and access (although out of the reach of children) to ensure that you take them on a daily basis.

Tips for Kids

Vitamin D deficiency among infants and children is estimated to be between 12% and 24%, although some estimates are much higher. Vitamin D is essential for calcium absorption and adequate bone mineralization in children. In addition, studies show that supplementation of vitamin D in the first year of life is protective against type 1 diabetes, and normal vitamin D levels in pregnant mothers reduces the risk of wheezing and asthma in their children. The AAP recommends daily intake of 400 IU of vitamin D for infants and children.

Be aware that many daily vitamin supplements for children contain artificial colors and sweeteners to make them more appealing to kids. Use a whole food supplement that is free of these additives for your children as well as yourself.

Don't forget to continue your

January habit of drinking at least eight glasses of water per day (one-half of your weight in ounces of water per day),

February habit of eating seven to nine servings of fruit and vegetables per day,

March habit of replacing refined white foods with whole grains,

April habit of exercising for at least thirty minutes five times per week,

May habit of detoxifying your system daily,

June habit of sleeping for seven to eight hours each night,

July habit of eating early, eating often, and stopping before it's too late,

August habit of increasing omega-3 fatty acids in your diet,

September habit of sharing a home-cooked meal with your family at least five times per week,

October habit of reducing your media diet, and

November habit of practicing stress-reducing strategies.

References

Cancer Trends Progress Report—2009/2010 Update. National Cancer Institute: National Institutes of Health. http:// progressreport.cancer.gov/doc_detail.asp?pid=1&did=2007&c hid=71&coid=707&mid=#links

Catherine F. Casey, MD; David C. Slawson, Md; And Lindsey R. Neal, Md Vitamin D Supplementation in Infants, Children, and Adolescents *Am Fam Physician*. 2010; 81 (6): 745-748, 750

Michael F. Holick, Vitamin D: Extraskeletal Health Endocrinol Metab Clin N Am 39 (2010) 381-400

O'Shea, Timothy WHOLE FOOD VITAMINS: Ascorbic Acid is Not Vitamin C *http://www.whale.to/a/shea1.html*

Vanga, S., Good, M., Howard, P., Vacek, J. Role of Vitamin D in Cardiovascular Health. Am J Cardiol 2010; 106: 798-805

Searing, D., Leung, D. Vitamin D in Atopic Dermatitis, Asthma and Allergic Diseases Immunol Allergy Clin N Am 30 (2010) 397-409

Conclusion

So you've made it to the end. You have now equipped yourself with great information about how to experience incredible health. Have you gotten started?

Like most doctors, I went into medicine for one principal reason: to make sick people better. But over the years, I have been noticing that people are getting *sicker*. Almost every chronic disease is rising in prevalence. And the most disturbing to me as a pediatrician is the increase in chronic disease rates in *children*, which is closely linked to the rising rates of childhood obesity. These worrisome trends led me on a search for the root causes of all these illnesses, which I have learned are poor nutrition and toxic lifestyle habits that rob the body of its innate healing mechanisms.

Therefore, the strategies laid out in this book are not just for some people—they are for everybody. Our bodies all work the same way and need the same basic care. And if we give our bodies the proper fuel and proper care (physically, mentally, and spiritually), they will serve us well and will resist disease.

So don't miss the point! This "change one thing" journey is about a lot more than weight loss. It's about regaining our health so that we can be equipped to thrive in our life's purpose, having the vitality, energy, and clarity to perform at an incredible level. I know you want that for yourself and your family. Don't procrastinate. Get started today.

For more information, come visit my website at www.ahealthytomorrow.org and join the Change One Thing Challenge. I'll be glad to post your story or answer your questions.

Here's to your healthy tomorrow!

INDEX